GLOBAL PROFILES

DISEASE FIGHTERS SINCE 1950

Ray Spangenburg and Diane K. Moser

☑® Facts On File, Inc.

I 95
19
11-8-00

Disease Fighters Since 1950

Facts On File, Inc.
11 Penn Plaza
New York NY 10001

Library of Congress Cataloging-in-Publication Data

Spangenburg, Ray, 1939–
    Disease fighters since 1950 / by Ray Spangenburg and Diane K. Moser
      p.   cm. — (Global profiles)
    Includes bibliographical references and index.
    ISBN 0-8160-3319-6 (hbk. : alk. paper)
    1. Medical scientists—Biography. 2. Medical sciences—
History—20th century. I. Moser, Diane, 1944– . II. Title.
III. Series.
    R134.S58 1997
    610'.92'2—dc20   96-5571
    [B]

Facts On File books are available at special discounts when purchased in bulk quantities for businesses, associations, institutions or sales promotions. Please call our Special Sales Department in New York at (212) 967-8800 or (800) 322-8755.

Text design by Catherine Rincon Hyman
Cover design by Nora Wertz
Map by Dale Williams

Front cover photographs:
Rita Levi-Montalcini (© The Nobel Foundation); Sir Michael Anthony Epstein (courtesy of Sir Michael Anthony Epstein); Gertrude Belle Elion (Glaxo Wellcome); Susumu Tonegawa (Massachusetts Institute of Technology); Adetokunbo Lucas (© Sue Owrutsky); microorganic forms (© Telegraph Colour Library/FPG International).

Printed in the United States of America

MP FOF 10 9 8 7 6 5 4 3 2 1

This book is printed on acid-free paper.

In memory of
Dave Richardson,
good friend, fighter,
and writer to the last

Contents

Acknowledgments

Many people have generously helped us with this book—gathering photos from dusty files, sending e-mail and faxes across continents, making suggestions about content. To all of you, a heart-felt thanks, and especially to Dr. Ade Lucas and Sir Anthony Epstein for taking time from busy schedules to answer our queries and questions, to Sylviane Guesdon-Cayré of the Institut Pasteur for struggling with our fractured French and supplying excellent materials, to Barry Shell of the Great Canadian Scientists program for sharing his research materials, to Dr. Geffrey Mecaskey of the Edna McConnell Clark Foundation for brainstorming with us, and to Maureen Maloney of University College London Medical School for her calm reassurances across the miles. And finally, to Nicole Bowen, our former editor at Facts On File, who conceived the project and helped us shape its genesis; and to Emily Ross and Hilary Poole, who brought it to conclusion.

Introduction

The story of science—and those who do science—is like a great adventure story and mystery rolled into one. It's the story of the search for answers, for pieces of the puzzle that forms the whole picture we long to see. Sometimes the work is tedious and requires long hours, but the promise of new information lures, and when a breakthrough comes, the joy is immense.

The story of science in the fight against disease has an added urgency: It is a race against time to save human lives. The tragedy of this fight is that there are always those for whom a discovery comes too late. And the irony is that as soon as one disease is vanquished, it seems, another rears its ugly head.

By the middle of the 20th century, the world seemed almost safe from infectious disease. Smallpox, polio, diphtheria, whooping cough, and yellow fever had been conquered or soon would be. Before long, tuberculosis had become a relic of 19th-century novels. The bubonic plague had wiped out one third to one half the population of England in the 14th century and a million people in northern Italy in two years in the 18th century. Now it seemed so distant from contemporary reality that it had taken on the aura of myth. Then along came AIDS in the 1980s, a disease we still don't know how to fight completely. And in 1995 came an outbreak of the Ebola virus, which took us by surprise, but burned itself out, for the moment.

For thousands of years, human beings have been struggling against the destructive ravages of disease, against forces that take power over their bodies to kill and maim and cause pain. Those who fight against these forces have always held a position of special respect in societies all over the world—both ancient and modern. These are the men and women who intervene to help humanity fight pain, infirmity, and untimely death.

Since 1950, we have seen many triumphs in their fight. By the 1970s poliomyelitis, rabies, and leprosy had all been brought under control. The years between 1940 and 1970 brought a dramatic drop in the cancer mortality rate, thanks to improvements in surgical techniques, radiation, and chemotherapy. We found out how to graft new skin on burn victims and transplant organs from unrelated donors. We developed drugs that helped our bodies fight leukemia and herpes. New technologies—such as the pacemaker, tomography, and dialysis—provided new methods of treatment and diagnosis. Identification of the genes that cause some genetic diseases, such as cystic fibrosis, has raised the hope that a cure or relief may be just around the corner. Isolation of the AIDS virus may help researchers find a vaccine or cure.

Despite the evidence at first glance, progress has continued in giant steps in the second half of the 20th century. By 1979, the World Health Organization (WHO) could proudly announce the successful worldwide eradication of smallpox. Perhaps most important was the new understanding, fostered by WHO, of international health concerns—and an implementation of social programs to begin taking the fight to the global level.

But, while the 20th century has brought exciting new technology and insights, it has also brought many unexpected challenges, including the frightening new disease called AIDS, ongoing struggles against the ravages of tropical diseases, and the continuing threats of cancer and heart disease. The fight is by no means won.

This book chronicles the stories of some of the great fighters for worldwide health in our time—stories of scientists and physicians at work, of men and women engaged in the detective work of finding out what causes disease, discovering new methods of diagnosing and new therapies for treating ailments, and looking for more effective means of preventing illness.

In this book, we'll follow the steps of Ade Lucas in his work with the World Health Organization and the World Bank; of Françoise Barré-Sinoussi of the Pasteur Institute in Paris as she searches for a cure for AIDS, the greatest public health concern since the great tuberculosis epidemics of the early 1900s; of Jonas Salk and Albert Sabin in their successful campaign against poliomyelitis; of Gertrude Elion as she searches for new drugs to combat cancer; of Bernard Kouchner in his activism to bring medical aid to disaster-stricken areas; and others.

These are the stories of today's disease fighters, the men and women who continue the fight that often seems, like the mythological hydra, to sprout new challenges for every apparent victory. These are some of their stories—exciting stories of the search for knowledge about disease. In telling them, we hope to challenge our readers to join their ranks—either in spirit or in fact.

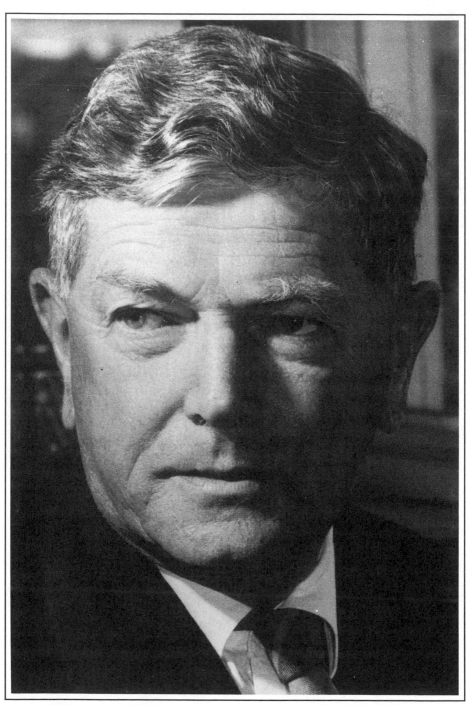

Sir Frank Macfarlane Burnet, 1960   (Copyright © The Nobel Foundation)

Sir Frank Macfarlane Burnet

THE ACQUISITION OF IMMUNOLOGICAL TOLERANCE (1899–1985)

> On the whole it was a happy unquestioning time when a normal boy's interest in birds' nests, yabbies and mussels in the creek, butterflies, or stones which might be valuable minerals, developed perhaps beyond the average level of enthusiasm and pertinacity in such things. It was fun "mucking about" along the creek . . .
>
> *Changing Patterns: An Atypical Autobiography*, 1969
> —Frank Macfarlane Burnet

As a boy growing up in rural Australia, Frank Macfarlane Burnet avidly explored the creek beds, watching the mud for signs of mussel valves, searching for a "white-eye's nest" and its blue-green eggs, catching whirligig beetles. He had a passion for beetles. Born September 3, 1899, in Traralgon, Victoria, he was the son of a local bank manager, Frank Burnet. His mother was the former Hadassah Pollock MacKay. When the boy was 10, they moved to Terang, another small town by a lake, where Burnet continued to pursue his interest in nature, watching birds, catching butterflies, and most of all, collecting beetles.

At Geelong College, in Geelong, Victoria, where he majored in biology and medicine, Burnet continued collecting beetles. When he continued his education in 1917 at Ormond College of the University of Melbourne, he went right on collecting beetles. He received his bachelor of science degree in 1922, followed a year later by his M.D. degree, after which he gained a dual appointment as resident pathologist at the Royal Melbourne Hospital and as researcher at the University of Melbourne's Walter and Eliza Hall Institute for Medical Research. He set the stage then for his two lifelong loves—clinical medical work and research.

Science, Burnet liked to say, was just creeping into medicine in the 1920s, when he began his study of medicine. But even though doctors could do very little for their patients, Burnet took great joy in what he called "the all-absorbing satisfaction of the clinical study of disease in its human setting." He cared about human pain.

"My attitude to the beetles, which it must be remembered was significant until I was over thirty, showed a steady progress toward sophistication."

—Frank Macfarlane Burnet in *Changing Patterns*, 1969

Insulin had been discovered, but was not yet available, and Burnet recalled commiserating with a young patient for whom he prescribed a diet of "5 per cent vegetables" (or their equivalent in sugar content). The boy became so depressed by the wretchedness of his food that he checked himself out of the hospital—with Burnet hoping that insulin would become available in time to save him.

During these years he wrote a science fiction story, which he submitted to the medical school magazine, *Speculum*. The theme, he later explained, was simple. In the distant future (1950 seemed a long way off at the time) medical training would consist of connecting each student to a current patient in such a way that the student could actually feel all the bodily sensations of the sick person. "No more struggles to interpret 'It's an awful shooting pain, doctor,' or 'it's a sort of funny turn,'" Burnet explained. The student would feel it all. Of course, the fictitious medical students hated this training so much that they had to be drafted into medical school. The editor of *Speculum* declined to publish it.

In 1926 a Beit Memorial fellowship enabled Burnet to travel to London to spend a year in residence at the Lister Institute of Preventive Medicine. There he earned his Ph.D. working with viruses and bacteriophages (in a way he was still collecting "bugs," just much smaller ones). On his return to Australia, he became assistant director of the Walter and Eliza Hall Institute in 1928. He would spend the next 37 years of his life at this institution, becoming director in early 1944.

As an experimentalist, Burnet became best known for developing methods of propagating viruses in chick embryos and for his work on the bacteriophage. The bacteriophage, or phage, a type of parasite that lives off viruses, was first discovered independently by British researcher Frederick W. Twort, in 1915, and French-Canadian scientist Félix H. d'Hérelle, in 1917. Since that time, phages have become useful for studying a wide range of topics in genetics and molecular biology, especially since the 1940s.

During the 1930s, while working on influenza with the virology unit of the Medical Research Council in London, Burnet found that flu virus could be grown in hen's eggs. From 1933 on, Burnet used the chick embryo in ovo (in the egg) as a means of cultivating and studying viruses, and he developed a special technique—for which he became famous—for inserting a virus into the embryo. Because he was working so closely with embryos, he became intrigued by the embryo's special character: First, it seemed to have no ability

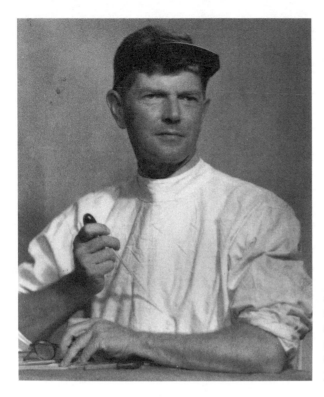

Burnet holding a pipette of the type he used for his work with chick embryos (Frank Macfarlane Burnet Collection, University of Melbourne Archives)

to resist a viral infection. Second, it also did not produce antibodies against viruses. In the process he found clues that led to breakthrough work in 1949 and the 1950s on the development of antibodies.

Burnet's thinking about antibodies was stimulated by two observations made by other researchers. First, E. Traub, working at the Rockefeller Institute, discovered a particular mouse virus that could infect the young while still in the uterus, without harming the infant mouse. Everything about the mouse developed normally, except that for the rest of its life, it would carry large amounts of the virus in all its tissues.

Meanwhile, in 1946 in Wisconsin, Ray Owen performed an interesting experiment in immunology. He showed that twin calves could share blood of mixed types (A, B, AB, O), interchanging blood through common circulation via the placenta surrounding them before birth. In this situation, the calves maintained the same mixture of genetically distinct blood types throughout their lives.

In both cases—Traub's mouse virus and Owen's mixed blood types—an adult body would have identified the foreign body as an antigen and would have produced an immune response.

As a result of his thinking about these examples, Burnet began to develop some ideas about how an individual's immune system distinguishes between self and nonself. For example, if you introduce an animal's red blood cells into another animal of another species, or even of the same species, why do antibodies develop—when the presence of these blood cells in the animal's own system doesn't produce antibodies?

Obviously, if an animal's cells destroy its own cells, something's going wrong. But Burnet's question was: What mechanism enables cells to recognize other cells that are different and yet part of the same organism? How do they know what to destroy and what not to destroy? Burnet went on in the 1950s to develop a theory to explain how antibodies are so quickly produced by an organism to fight off antigens never before encountered. In his laboratory, Burnet used a chick embryo to try artificially to produce tolerance against standard antigens. But the experiments failed. However, Peter Medawar (in the next chapter) took up the experimental work where Burnet left off.

Burnet extended his theories about the "self-and-nonself" prob-

"When I was taught bacteriology in 1920, only two virus diseases were mentioned, rabies and smallpox with its cowpox variant . . . In 1966, . . . some two hundred distinguishable types of virus had been isolated from human material . . ."

—Frank Macfarlane Burnet in *Changing Patterns*, 1969

lem of immunology to develop what he called the "clonal selection theory of immunity." This theory, though controversial, has stimulated a great deal of experimental work with important results for both general biology and practical surgery and medicine.

As we'll see, Burnet's predictions concerning the ability of the body to accept transplanted tissue were confirmed in graftings conducted by Medawar on embryonic rats inoculated with foreign tissue. For his work on the acquisition of the immunological tolerance necessary for organ transplantation, Burnet shared the 1960 Nobel Prize in physiology or medicine with Peter Medawar.

A prolific writer of books on science and medicine, Burnet wrote numerous books for nonscientists, including: *Immunology, Aging, and Cancer*, 1976. He was elected to the prestigious Royal Society of London in 1942 and received the Society's Royal Medal in 1947 and the Copley Medal in 1959. In 1954 he was elected a foreign associate of the U.S. National Academy of Sciences. In 1951 he was knighted. Frank Macfarlane Burnet died August 31, 1985. He is the only Australian ever to receive the Nobel Prize in physiology or medicine.

Chronology

September 3, 1899	Frank Macfarlane Burnet born in Traralgon, Victoria, Australia
1922	Receives bachelor of science degree from the University of Melbourne
1923	Receives M.D. degree from Melbourne
1926	Journeys to London for a year in residence at the Lister Institute of Preventive Medicine (Ph.D. 1928)

1928	After returning to Australia, Burnet marries Edith Linda Druce
1932–33	Burnet becomes a Rockefeller fellow at London's National Institute for Medical Research
1947	Elected a member of the Royal Society in London
1951	Knighted by King George V of England
1960	Nobel Prize (shared with Medawar)
1973	Edith Burnet dies
1974	Burnet marries Hazel Jenkin
August 31, 1985	Burnet dies in Melbourne

Further Reading

Burnet, Sir Macfarlane. *Changing Patterns: An Atypical Autobiography.* New York: American Elsevier Publishing Company, Inc., 1969. Burnet gives a thoroughly delightful overview of his professional life and work.

Daintith, John, et al., eds. *Biographical Encyclopedia of Scientists, 2nd Edition.* Vol. 1, pp. 131–132. Bristol: Institute of Physics Publishing, 1994.

McGraw-Hill Modern Men of Science, pp. 81–82. New York: McGraw-Hill, 1966.

Nelson, R. *Virus Hunter in Australia.* Melbourne: Nelson, 1966. Difficult to find, this is the only full-length biography available on Burnet.

Newton, David E. "Frank Macfarlane Burnet, 1899–1985," in *Notable Twentieth-Century Scientists*, edited by Emily J. McMurray, Vol. I, pp. 281–283. New York: Gale Research, Inc., 1995.

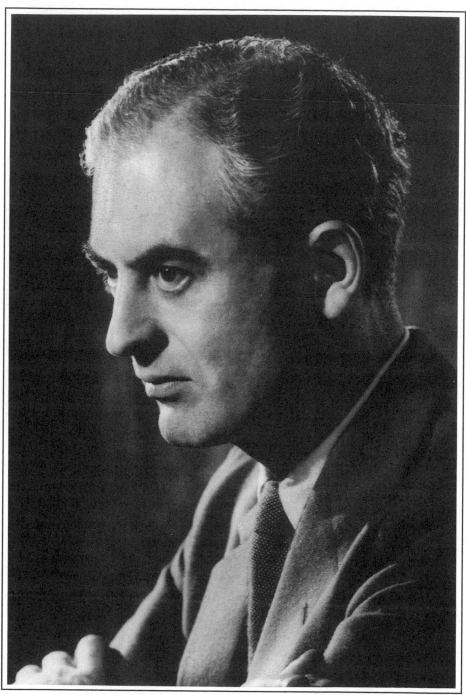

Peter Brian Medawar, 1960   (Copyright © The Nobel Foundation)

Sir Peter Medawar

PAVING THE WAY FOR ORGAN TRANSPLANTS (1915–1987)

The year was 1940, and England was at war with Germany. The word had gone out in the town of Oxford: Be prepared for low-flying enemy German bombers at any time, even in daylight. Many families who could afford to had already sent wives and children north or across the Atlantic to safety. But Peter Medawar [MED uh wahr] was working on experiments on the effect of wounds and deep burns on skin, and so he had stayed at his laboratory in Oxford; he and his wife, Jean, who was also a zoologist, had decided they would keep their family together.

One sunny day, Peter was reading in the backyard of their little house. Jean was tending the garden, and their daughter was playing nearby. Suddenly, a shadow fell across the sun and the heavens seemed to open up with a resounding roar. They could see the low-flying plane through the birch trees at the end of the garden as they scooped up their daughter and raced for their air raid shelter, barely arriving before the earth shook with a dull thud. When the air cleared, the young zoologists found out the plane had not been an enemy, after all. It was a British plane gone out of control, and one young airman was desperately injured, with 67 percent of his body seared with third-degree burns—that is, burns damaging the entire thickness of his skin.

What Peter Medawar thought of as his "messing about" days in his laboratory had come to an end—the small intellectual exercises he had always tinkered with were shoved aside. Now he had a real and crucial challenge before him, with a human being waiting for the answers: Could he find a way to graft new skin over this man's massive burns?

Peter Brian Medawar was born February 28, 1915, in Petropolis, a suburb of Rio de Janeiro, Brazil, and he retained dual Brazilian and British citizenship throughout his life. His father, Nicholas Medawar, was from Lebanon, the modern site of ancient Phoenicia. "Like many Phoenicians before him," Peter Medawar wrote in his autobiography, "my father left Jounieh, his birthplace in the Lebanon, and traveled west in search of his fortune." His first stop was London, where he met and fell in love with Muriel Dowling, whom later he married. Nicholas became a sales agent in Rio de Janeiro for a British manufacturer of dental supplies.

Although Peter and his brother Philip spent their early years in Brazil, they attended boarding schools in England, spending holidays and vacations with relatives. Peter hated the regimentation and pretension of the schools he attended, but he had one unusually good teacher—a science teacher—who brought out his intelligence and imaginative ability. He

"Like many Phoenicians before him, my father left Jounieh, his birthplace in the Lebanon, and traveled west in search of his fortune."

—Peter Medawar in *Memoir of a Thinking Radish*, 1986

attended Magdalen College, Oxford, and had the good luck in the one-teacher-one-student tradition of the university to draw an excellent tutor. "A good tutor," he explained in his autobiography, *Memoir of a Thinking Radish*, "will excite enough respect to cause his student to want to please him and earn his praise, and will be most anxious to bring out his student's every capability and help him to get as good a degree as he is capable of." In addition to zoology, Medawar pursued an interest in philosophy at Oxford, and his many writings on the philosophy and practice of science provide witty, imaginative and thoughtful insights into the workings of a fine mind.

Medawar graduated from Oxford in 1937, but remained there to work under Howard Florey, the co-discoverer of penicillin. In Florey's laboratory he began a series of experiments related to war wounds, especially burns.

Because Medawar was already known for his work with burns, authorities asked him to see if he could help the severely burned airman who nearly crashed in Medawar's backyard. He visited the man in the hospital, and what he saw there shook him. "If a burnt patient could be kept alive through the acute stage of a burn," as this man had, he later explained, "the dead tissues would be sloughed and leave in their place a raw area filled with a spongy red tissue of repair called 'granulation tissue' through which there was a constant seepage of body fluid."

What the man needed was a new skin. But how? Surgeons had sometimes succeeded in grafting skin from one site to another on the same person. But this man didn't have enough of his own skin left to provide material for grafting. In the past, every effort to graft skin from one person to another had always failed, although no one knew why. Did the body discriminate between its own cells and other living cells? How can it tell the difference between what Macfarlane Burnet called Self and Non-Self? Medawar now poured all his time and energy and thought into finding answers to this question.

He began to think about how to make the skin that was left do the job for the whole body, even though not a lot was left. He tried growing a tissue culture from some small pieces of skin, left over from plastic surgery, to see if they would increase in size. He tried "harvesting" epidermal cells, by plucking them from outer layers of skin, and then making a sort of soup that he spread over the raw area. And he tried laying some ultra-thin slices of skin on the surface of the wound.

None of this worked. He found that only the full thickness of skin would work—otherwise the wound contracted, forming deep, disfiguring scars that sometimes even prevented free movement. A surgeon from Spain, P. Gabarro, finally came up with an idea that worked: a series of "postage stamp" grafts—small pieces of skin whose cells gradually spread out to cover the areas in between. The airman recovered and in 1988 he was living in Canada raising Alsatian dogs.

Medawar kept pursuing the question, though. Skin grafts from a donor would be the easiest, the best answer, but these were never successful. Why? If you could do blood transfusions without rejection, why couldn't you graft skin from one person to another? He obtained a grant to work in the Burns Unit of the Glasgow Royal Infirmary in Scotland. There he would have both patients and facilities for research. Working with an assistant, Medawar decided to find out exactly what happened inside a graft from a donor (called a homograft) that was different from what went on inside a graft from oneself (an autograft).

They worked with a patient, Mrs. McK., whose entire back had been burned when she had fallen on a gas stove. From her brother, who had volunteered to be a donor, they took a series of pinch grafts, which they placed in a row on her back. Then they placed a parallel row of autografts from her own skin. They examined the two rows of grafts daily, both observationally and under a microscope. The microscope work told the tale, but extracting the story wasn't easy. For each microscope slide Medawar took samples, which he then impregnated with wax, sliced, stained, and then examined. The first few days showed little difference between the homograft row and the autograft row. But then in the homografts he began to notice a steady invasion of lymphocytes—the white blood cells that form the front line of attack against foreign invaders. In about 10 days, these grafts were rejected and fell off. The others stayed. Now he had an answer: Skin grafts from another individual of the same species were rejected because the body mounted an immunological attack on them.

This work, out of which a great deal more work followed, and which paved the way for organ transplants, was the basic discovery for which Peter Medawar received the Nobel Prize 15 years later (with Macfarlane Burnet) in 1960.

In 1944, on his return from the Burns Unit, Medawar became a senior research fellow at St. Johns College, Oxford, and university demonstrator in zoology and comparative anatomy until 1947, when he became the chair of zoology at Birmingham University.

At Birmingham, he formed a research team with two of his graduate students, Rupert Everett "Bill" Billingham and Leslie Brent. Together they explored an issue raised when Medawar attended an International Congress of Genetics at Stockholm in 1948. He promised another investigator, Hugh Donald, that he could come up with a foolproof method for distinguishing identical from fraternal twin calves. He thought that identical twin calves would accept a skin graft from each other, while fraternal twins would not: that is, because identical twins come from a single egg, they would have a mutual tolerance that the others would not. However, to the surprise of Medawar's research team, the calves accepted skin grafts from their twins regardless of their identical or fraternal origin.

Not until they saw the work of Macfarlane Burnet at the University of Melbourne and Ray D. Owen, who was now at California Institute of Technology, did they realize why. Because blood transfuses through the placenta between twins in cattle whether they are identical or not, the calves acquire an immunological tolerance for each other before they are born. This meant that the body does not recognize tissue as alien if exposed at a very early age.

Medawar's new insights led to further experiments to discover the mechanisms of graft rejection and ways of suppressing the immune response in surgical grafting and organ transplants. If the immune reaction was suppressed while the skin grafts or organ grafts were settling into their new home, could this type of surgery succeed? He pursued this question, injecting tissue cells from adult mice into developing mice embryos—and in 1953 discovered that the younger mice tolerated the grafting. He had discovered acquired immunological tolerance, the ability of an organism to overcome its normal tendency to reject foreign tissue and/or organs.

"My mind always goes blank when I'm asked why did I get a Nobel Prize, or how did I get it?"

—Peter Medawar in *The Threat and the Glory*, 1959

In 1951, when he became professor of zoology at University College, London, he took his research team, Billingham and Brent, with him, and in 1960, when he and Burnet shared the Nobel Prize, he shared the prize money with his team.

In 1962 Medawar was named director of the National Institute for Medical Research, London, a key post in the British scientific world. He later wrote that he left University

College reluctantly, because he knew he would have no students at "Mill Hill," as the National Institute was called. But the idea of directing an institution free from funding hassles and focused as "Mill Hill" attracted him. Unfortunately, the job entailed a very heavy administrative load, with extensive transatlantic travel, and Medawar stubbornly refused to cut back on his research. Although he had many warning signs of high blood pressure, he continued to push hard and work long hours until 1969 when he suffered a massive stroke that left him partially paralyzed. He continued as director until 1971, continuing his research, but only at half-capacity.

After 1969, Medawar continued research he had begun on cancer at the Clinical Research Centre in London. A second stroke, though, in 1980 and a third in 1984 impaired him further, but he continued writing. The books he wrote during this period include *Induction and Intuition in Scientific Thought* (1969), *Advice to a Young Scientist* (1979), and *Memoir of a Thinking Radish* (1986). In a touching salute near the end of his *Memoir*, Medawar pays tribute to his wife, Jean, whom he met at Oxford and married in 1937. They co-authored several books, and he clearly considered her his best friend and closest companion, quipping that an unexpectedly happy consequence of his illness was that he no longer ever went anywhere without her.

Medawar received the Royal Medal from the Royal Society in 1959 and was knighted in 1965. Although he completed the requirements for a doctorate at Oxford, he felt the fee for the degree was an unnecessary expense and never paid it. So he enjoyed joking that instead he was collecting honorary doctorates from A to Z. The list of universities paying him this tribute is lengthy, ranging from the University of Alberta to Washington University in both St. Louis and Seattle, and accounting for most of the alphabet in between.

He admitted that Exeter was cheating for X and that Yale and Zimbabwe had not come through.

Of his Nobel work, he wrote in *Memoir of a Thinking Radish* that "the ultimate importance of the discovery of tolerance turned out to be not practical, but moral. It put new heart into the many biologists and surgeons who were working to make it possible to graft, for example, kidneys from one person to another." In the world of biomedical research this sort of hope is at the heart of it all. Peter Medawar died on October 2, 1987.

Chronology

February 28, 1915	Born near Rio de Janeiro, Brazil
1919	Medawar comes to England
1932	Enters Magdalen College, Oxford
1935	Receives bachelor's degree, Oxford; begins graduate work under Howard W. Florey
1937	Marries Jean Shinglewood Taylor, a zoologist
1940	Works on severely burned patients at the Glasgow Royal Infirmary, Scotland
1947	Becomes professor of zoology at the University of Birmingham
1949	Elected to the Royal Society
1960	Nobel Prize (shared with Burnet)
1965	Medawar is knighted
1969	Publication of *Induction and Intuition in Scientific Thought*
1979	Publication of *Advice to a Young Scientist*

| 1986 | Publication of *Memoir of a Thinking Radish* |
| October 2, 1987 | Medawar dies |

Further Reading

Medawar, Jean. *A Very Decided Preference*. New York: W.W. Norton, 1990. Biography of Medawar written by his wife. Tells the particularly poignant story of Medawar's drive to continue working despite a crippling stroke in 1969.

Medawar, Peter. *Advice to a Young Scientist*. New York: Harper, 1979.

———. "Immunological Tolerance," in *Nobel Lectures*. Nobel Foundation, 1964, pp. 704–715.

———. *Memoir of a Thinking Radish: An Autobiography*. Oxford: Oxford University Press, 1986.

———. "My Life in Science (1966)," in *The Threat and the Glory: Reflections on Science and Scientists*. New York: HarperCollins, 1990. The transcript of a BBC program interview, originally broadcast on April 25, 1966.

Mertz, Leslie. "Peter Brian Medawar, 1915–1987," *Notable Twentieth-Century Scientists*, edited by Emily J. McMurray, Vol. I, pp. 1353–1356. New York: Gale Research, Inc., 1995.

Mitchison, N. A. "Sir Peter Medawar (1915–1987)." *Nature*, November 12, 1987, p. 112.

"Sir Peter Medawar." *New Scientist*, April 12, 1984, pp. 14–20.

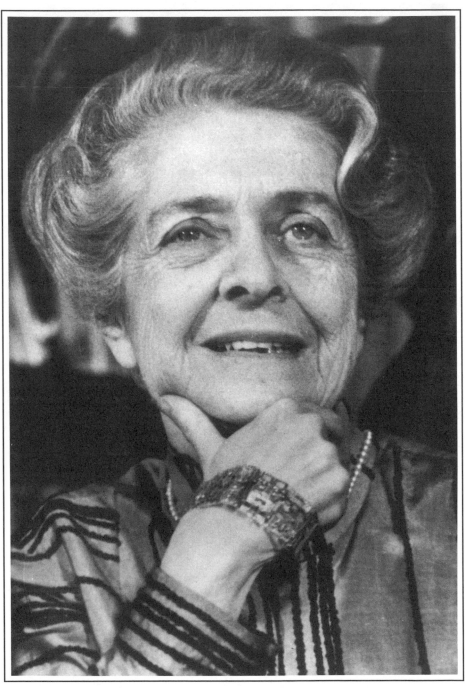

Rita Levi-Montalcini, 1986 (Copyright © The Nobel Foundation)

Rita Levi-Montalcini

"UNDERESTIMATING OBSTACLES" AND THE NERVE GROWTH FACTOR (1909–)

Rita Levi-Montalcini's [LEE vee mon tal CHEE nee] bedroom had taken on a very unusual look in 1941. Where most people would expect to find a table with flowers basking in the filtered mountain sunlight of northern Italy, Levi-Montalcini had an egg incubator, built out of scraps and odds and ends by her brother, Gino, an architect. Nearby she kept her stereomicroscope; in another corner her prized binocular Zeiss microscope. The windows were shuttered and darkened. At the door, her mother protected her from interruption. "You can't go in," she would warn. "She's operating."

Prohibited by fascist law from practicing medicine or conducting university research because she was Jewish, here the young physician had found a way to continue working—without salary or fees, yet repaid in the knowledge that her work stood on the cutting edge of her field.

It was the early years of World War II, and under the dictatorship of the fascist leader Benito Mussolini, Italy had begun following the lead of Nazi Germany as early as 1936. Under pressure from Adolf Hitler, Italy by

1939 had also passed anti-Semitic laws similar to those passed in Germany. The situation had become dangerous—not only for Levi-Montalcini, but for her patients—for her even to pay house calls. Thus, despite a recent completion of her medical degree, Rita Levi-Montalcini's career as a physician had ended almost as soon as it had begun.

The war drew closer each day, but on quiet days, when the shelling stopped, Levi-Montalcini would make her tour to the neighboring farms on her bicycle, collecting eggs. She needed fertile eggs, she explained, because they were "better for the children" (although she had no children—she needed the chick embryos to find the answers she sought in her bedroom lab).

At home, she would remove the portions she needed for her experiments, and then, to her brother Gino's horror, scramble the remainder for the family breakfast. When the shelling was too close, she would grab her priceless Zeiss microscope and rush with the others to the bomb shelter.

Under these inhospitable circumstances, Rita Levi-Montalcini bravely and stubbornly began the work that would one day earn her the Nobel Prize in physiology or medicine.

Rita Levi-Montalcini and her twin sister Paola were born April 22, 1909, in the city of Turin within view of the snowcapped Alps of northern Italy. The twins, Rita and Paola, were the youngest of four children—their brother, Gino, was seven years their senior, and their sister, Anna, five years. Adamo Levi, their father, was an electrical engineer who had built an ice factory on the outskirts of Turin; he considered the factory a great technological advance, however unpopular he was with those who made an easy living collecting ice from the mountains, keeping it in cool underground cellars to sell in the summer.

Levi-Montalcini characterizes her family as Victorian in spirit; her father (known affectionately to his sisters as Damino the Terrible), made all the decisions, and her mother, Adele Montalcini, went calmly along with them. "I was brought up in an environment," she wrote in her autobiography, *In Praise of Imperfection*, "that, though not permissive, was brimming with affection and never troubled by disagreements between my mother and father." But several years later, she told a journalist, "It was a very patriarchal society, and I simply resented, from early childhood, that women were reared in such a way that everything was decided by the man."

Levi-Montalcini felt a vivid affection for her mother, whose supportive warmth saw her through the common traumas of childhood. Yet, unlike her twin Paola, Rita always felt distant from her father, to his disappointment and her own regret after his death. She later realized that from him she had inherited her inquisitive mind and her seriousness and dedication to work. She came to share his secular philosophy and love of the intellectual life, and she admired the tenacity, energy, and ingenuity that had enabled him to overcome obstacles and pursue his visions. Unfortunately, before she could overcome the communication barriers between them, he died just after she and Paola turned 23.

As twins often do, Rita and Paola grew up even more closely allied than most brothers and sisters. Gino and Anna "came into the category of third parties." Yet the twins were very different. Paola showed an artistic talent from an early age, which she shared with her brother. (Paola would later become a fine artist; and Gino, an architect.) With her sister Anna (known as Nina), Rita shared literary interests—especially English novels such as Emily Brontë's *Wuthering Heights* and Virginia Woolf's *To the Lighthouse*. But like her father, Rita found her greatest gifts in the arena of mathematics and science.

Clearly not identical in talents, Paola and Rita didn't resemble each other physically or temperamentally either. Paola had laughing blue eyes, a cheery, sparkling demeanor, and—at least as a child—closely resembled her father. Rita looked more like her mother's mother, with gray-green eyes, a melancholic gaze, and a love of solitude.

As a child, Rita noticed an uneasiness in her middle-class neighborhood about her religion. Friends at her playground seemed curious and anxious to classify her. But her father, who was a non-practicing Jew, advised her to avoid being pigeon-holed: "You children are freethinkers," he said. "When you reach twenty-one, you'll decide whether you wish to continue as before or whether you prefer to belong to the Jewish or Catholic faith. But don't worry about it. If you are asked, you should answer that you are a freethinker." And so she did.

Adamo Levi's opinion about the place of education for women, however, was less than enlightened. He saw no reason why a woman needed a university education. Of his children, only Gino, the son, attended a college preparatory school; the girls attended a finishing school. Their aunts, Levi reasoned, had seen nothing but grief in their marriages, which he attributed to false expectations bestowed upon them by their university education. For Paola, who planned (and successfully pursued) a career in painting and sculpture, the choice did no great damage. But when Rita graduated from secondary school at age 18, she was blocked from any intellectual career, especially in the sciences, because the school had given her no preparation to enter college. When she sadly watched her governess die of cancer three years later, she resolved to become a physician and pursued the issue with her father. Finally, he consented to let her prepare for the entrance exams and provided for tutoring for her—but only if she would promise never to marry. Education and family life for a woman, he was convinced, did not mix. But Rita knew her mind and agreed to the proposition without regret.

Levi-Montalcini passed the entrance exams with distinction and in 1930 she enrolled in the Turin School of Medicine. There she organized study groups in the library and presented an intensely studious demeanor in the laboratories and lecture halls. She studied under Giuseppe Levi (no relation to her father), a well-known histologist and embryologist with a resolute and imperious manner—coincidentally much like her father's—and a boundless energy that knew no obstacles. Also like her father, he was inclined toward fits of rage. But he was a fine scientist and gave her a strong background for the work she would eventually do. She received her degree in 1939, and for a short time worked as Levi's assistant.

But shortly after she received her medical degree, the curtain closed on all professional work for Jews in Italy. What was to be an exciting new beginning seemed instead to be an abrupt and unjust termination of all possibilities. Europe was in the throes of one of the ugliest periods of recent history. In Germany, Adolf Hitler had led his nation to war against the rest of western Europe and promoted hatred against the Jews. Concentration camp deaths that would number in the millions had already begun. In Italy, Benito Mussolini had become Hitler's ally and followed in his footsteps. Soon the anti-Semitic laws in Italy forced Levi-Montalcini to leave the university. For a brief time, she went to Belgium, where she was offered a position at the Neurological Institute in Brussels, but by this time German troops began to invade Belgium. As the dangers worsened, Rita also began to fear for the safety of her family in Italy. Levi-Montalcini returned home, depressed and dejected. Because of the laws, she couldn't practice medicine, use the university library or even visit friends at the university. She sat idly, day after day, time hanging in the air like a cobweb.

Then one autumn day, a friend, Rodolfo Amprimo, stopped by to visit. "One doesn't lose heart in the face of first difficulties," he scolded her brusquely when he found out she had stopped working. You could set up a small laboratory, he insisted. You could work. She agreed, and set up the secret laboratory in her bedroom. It was the beginning of Rita Levi-Montalcini's journey into what she later called "the jungle," the vast tangle of the nervous system with its billions of cells.

She chose a project that would be easy to do under these strained circumstances. She had read a paper by Viktor Hamburger, a pioneer in nerve development. As she thought about it, she thought of an experiment that she could pursue

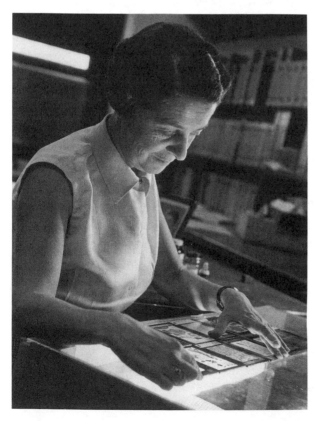

Levi-Montalcini checking over her slides
(Photo by Herb Weitman, courtesy of Washington University, St. Louis)

with chicken embryos. Fertilized chicken eggs were easy to obtain, and Gino could build her an incubator—a glass thermo-regulated box with two circular openings for arms—to develop the chick embryos in. In addition to her microscopes, her laboratory tools consisted of a few watch-makers' forceps, ophthalmic microscissors, and sewing needles ground down to serve as tiny scalpels and spatulas.

Before long, Giuseppe Levi heard about her project and, since he also had been purged from his professional position, he joined her in her tiny laboratory, the size of a convent cell. As in a convent, here she was able to shut out the world and its atrocities and focus on her work. She wandered in the jungle of nerve endings and shut out the human jungle beyond her bedroom door.

She was studying the mysteries of very early-stage embryonic development—trying to understand the mechanism by which cells develop and differentiate in the spinal cord at the very beginning of life. She had conceived an experiment that could add to the base of knowledge in this area: to excise tissues in the limbs that had not yet been reached by the developing network of nerves and then observe how the absence of these cells affected the development of the motor cells in the spinal cord and sensory cells in the dorsal root ganglia (bundles of nerve fibers). Little did she know that she was making the first steps toward an important discovery—one that would eventually win her the Nobel Prize. During the years 1941–43, Levi-Montalcini lived in a country cottage in the Piedmont region of Italy. But when the Germans began the invasion of Italy, she and her family escaped to Florence, where she continued to live in hiding until the Allied liberation of Italy in 1944.

Levi-Montalcini felt that she never experienced the degree of prejudice in Italy that ran rampant in Germany during the years that followed. Yet, because of the discriminatory laws passed in 1938, she couldn't publish her papers in Italian journals. So she published her papers in Swiss and Belgian journals, which may have worked to her advantage since she received international attention that she might not have received with Italian publication. In fact, she discovered, she had readers in the United States, including Viktor Hamburger, who had fled Germany and was by this time at Washington University in St. Louis.

In 1945, after the war, Levi-Montalcini worked for several months in the hospitals, caring for wounded soldiers and civilians, but then she returned to her laboratory at the University of Turin, where she continued her previous work. Then one day in 1946, she received a letter from Washington University in St. Louis. It was from Viktor Hamburger, now the chair of the department of zoology, who had read her work. Would she come, he asked, and work for six months on a problem related to her experiments? Levi-Montalcini couldn't pass it up. In 1947 she left Italy by boat for the United States. For the first time in years, opportunity seemed to spread before her.

When she arrived in St. Louis, she was delighted by the open, park-like campus shaded by trees. But the student behavior amazed her. Groups of students sprawled on the lawns with their books—in Turin no one would ever have been allowed to set foot on the grass. In the classrooms, their manner was casual and the women sat knitting during lectures.

Hamburger was cordial and set her up with lab space. He was interested in her work, it turned out, because it was so close to his, and yet seemed to be headed in a different direction. Both of them were looking at embryonic nerve tissue to see how it differentiated into specialized types. Hamburger held that differentiation of nerve cells depends on their destination. Based on his observations when he had excised limbs in growing embryos, he thought that an organizing factor, probably contained in the limb, was in effect "calling out" to the nerve cells in the spinal column. In a normal embryo, he hypothesized, the nerve cells respond to this call from the limbs. When the limb buds are excised, the call no longer goes out to the nerve cell and so the nerve cells don't specialize, and they don't grow away from the spinal cord.

But when Rita Levi-Montalcini had conducted similar experiments in her bedroom lab in Turin, she had reached a different conclusion. Yes, fewer nerve cells grew out toward the area where the limb bud used to be, but to her the evidence seemed to indicate that a nutrient was missing—some factor necessary to the development of the nerve cell that was normally produced by the limb. She saw evidence in her experiments that the nerve cell differentiation did take place, even though the limb was gone, but that the nerve cell quickly shriveled and died without the needed nutrient.

When she arrived in St. Louis, the plan was that she would stay six months. Instead she stayed 30 years, with frequent trips home to Italy to visit her family. Levi-Montalcini spent the next few years looking for the trophic factor that she had intuited during her war-time experiments. A former student of Hamburger's had shown that a certain mouse tumor cell line (sarcoma 180) caused more nerve cells to grow. Using this piece of information, Levi-Montalcini decided to see what would happen if she introduced cells from these tumors into the chick embryo. She noticed that something present in the tumor caused the nerve cells of the embryo to differentiate at a faster rate—and to produce more nerve cells. "These fiber bundles passed between the cells like rivulets of water flowing steadily over a bed of stones," she later recalled. But they weren't connected to the tumor cells. They were coming from the chick ganglia.

She began trying to find out what was causing this effect. Could the trophic factor be a fluid? The only way she could prove this hypothesis would be to perform an in vitro experiment. If she took a glass dish, placed a nerve ganglion in it with the tumor nearby—instead of placing the tumor cells in the embryo itself—and got the same effect, there could be little doubt that a fluid was at work.

The best place she knew to do in vitro work was in the lab of a friend who was working in Brazil. So, tucking a couple of tumor-carrying mice in her pocket with food to nibble on, she boarded a plane for Rio de Janeiro. But the experiments in Brazil went poorly at first. She placed bits of tumor from the two mice next to the chick ganglia as planned. Nothing happened, and her heart sank. In her letters to Hamburger she had no success to report. But for some reason she refused to give up. As she later wrote in her autobiography, *In Praise of Imperfection*, she possessed the knack of "underestimating the obstacles standing between me and what I want to accomplish—a trait I believe I inherited from my father." This trait, she believes, is one of the keys to her success as a scientist. Others might call it supreme perseverance.

Now she asked, What could be wrong? Maybe something in the tumor functioned as a toxin and stopped the growth. Maybe when the tumor was introduced into the chick it didn't produce this toxin. So she placed a piece of tumor that had been grown on a chick embryo side by side with the ganglia. And that was it! "A fibrullar halo," a dense array of fibers,

> "I landed at Rio de Janeiro airport on a stormy September afternoon in 1952. I was not alone: two little white mice were spying, with their pinpoint eyes, on whatever they could glimpse through the holes in the top of the small cardboard box that I had fitted into my overcoat pocket."
>
> —Levi-Montalcini, *In Praise of Imperfection*, 1988

spilled out around the ganglia. The Nobel committee in Sweden would later call her discovery a "fascinating example of how a skilled observer can create a concept out of apparent chaos."

Rita Levi-Montalcini flew back to St. Louis gleefully. When she arrived she was met by more good news. In her absence, Viktor Hamburger had found a young biochemist, Stanley Cohen, to work with her to isolate the trophic factor and identify nature and function. As they worked together over the coming years, they turned up other factors as well.

It took a lot of work, and for years little attention was paid to the factor Rita Levi-Montalcini had discovered, which she came to call the nerve growth factor, or NGF. Not a conventional hormone, this was a previously unknown type of molecule—one that is necessary for the development of a particular type of cell. Ultimately, Levi-Montalcini was able to show that this substance, NGF, plays a crucial role in the development of nerve cells and influences the orderly development of tissues. Levi-Montalcini also showed that growth factors of various kinds influence the development of different cell types within the body.

In the human body, nerve growth factor is produced by "target" cells in a wide variety of tissues. When it reaches a nerve cell, NGF binds to a receptor on the cell surface and is carried to the nerve cell nucleus. The chemical message it delivers prompts the cell to grow projections, or axons, that reach out toward the target cells, connecting with them and forming vast networks called synapses. In this way—by the nerve cells' growing toward target cells—an orderly network of nerves is created throughout the body.

In 1961, a U.S. National Science Foundation grant enabled Levi-Montalcini to set up a small research laboratory in Rome. This arrangement allowed her to spend more time with her family, alternating between Rome and St. Louis. Finally, after retiring from Washington University in 1981,

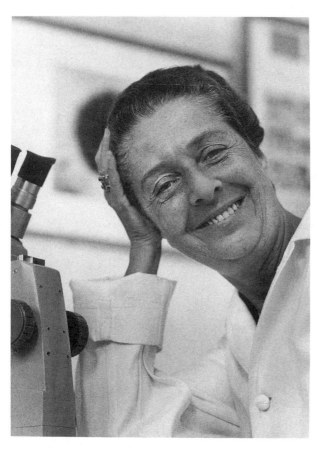

Taking a moment to look up from her work at Washington University, 1963
(Photo by Herb Weitman, courtesy of Washington University, St. Louis)

she moved to Rome, where she shares a double apartment with Paola.

Levi-Montalcini's research uncovered the existence of NGF and showed its effect on the development of sensory and sympathetic nerve cells, but much about it remains a mystery. Clearly, NGF is essential to the development of nerve cells. But what more can we find out about how it works and what uses it may have? Since Levi-Montalcini's discovery, further research has indicated that nerve growth factor also contributes to the survival and health mainte-nance of certain brain cells—among them, the cells that degenerate in Alzheimer's and Huntington's diseases. Does a lack of NGF contribute to the development of these two diseases? Levi-Montalcini's work may also prove useful in developing new methods for treatment of Parkinson's, a degenerative disease of the nervous system caused by a lack of dopamine, a particular neurotransmitter (substance that sends or inhibits nerve impulses at a synapse). Researchers hope that NGF may have the potential to revive damaged neurons, especially those damaged by diseases such as Alzheimer's. And, because of the importance of NGF during the development of the embryonic nervous system, Levi-Montalcini's research may also lead to a better understanding of certain birth defects. Nerve growth factor may also prove useful in healing damage to the peripheral nervous system found in those suffering from diabetes or undergoing chemotherapy.

Other growth factors have been found, and for these factors, researchers have discovered many applications to medicine. Growth factors are used to speed burn healing. They can reduce the side effects of chemotherapy and radiation therapy. And biotechnology research companies are exploring the possibility that still other growth factors may exist that could provide hope for regenerating motor neurons in damaged spinal-cord tissue.

In the 1980s it was found that oncogenes, cancer-causing genetic elements, carry a code for the manufacture of proteins that are similar in structure to growth factors and their receptors (chemical groupings on cell surfaces that bind to specific substances). This finding suggested that cancers may involve a failure in the regulation of growth factors.

In 1968 Rita Levi-Montalcini was elected to the U.S. National Academy of Sciences, and she is the only female member of the Papal Academy of Rome. In 1986 she shared the Nobel Prize in physiology or medicine with Stanley Cohen for their

"The moment you stop working, you are dead."

—Levi-Montalcini, 1993

work in the discovery and isolation of the nerve growth factor.

Now in her 80s, Levi-Montalcini is currently exploring the role of the nerve growth factor in the immune and endocrine systems. "The moment you stop working, you are dead," she exclaimed to one interviewer recently. "For me, it would be unhappiness beyond anything else."

Chronology

April 22, 1909	Rita Levi-Montalcini born (with her twin sister Paola) in Turin, Italy
1925	Constitutional government in Italy ends; Mussolini, as head of the fascist party, becomes dictator
1932	Rita's father, Adamo Levi, dies of heart failure
1936	Levi-Montalcini graduates with top honors from medical school
1938	Anti-Semitic laws are declared in Italy, severely limiting the civil liberties of Jews
1939	Leaves Italy to pursue research at the Neurological Institute in Brussels
1941	Rita and her brother Gino begin setting up her hidden laboratory at home
1947	At the invitation of Viktor Hamburger, Levi-Montalcini joins the department of zoology at Washington University in St. Louis, Missouri
1952	Travels to Rio de Janeiro to perform in vitro experiments; on return is joined in her research at Washington University by Stanley Cohen, a biochemist

1962	Levi-Montalcini returns to Italy on a part-time basis
1968	Elected to the U.S. National Academy of Sciences
1981	Levi-Montalcini opens her Cellular Biology Laboratory in Rome
1986	Rita Levi-Montalcini receives the Nobel Prize, with Stanley Cohen, for the work on the Nerve Growth Factor

Further Reading

Dash, Joan. *The Triumph of Discovery: Women Scientists Who Won the Nobel Prize*. Englewood Cliffs, NJ: Julian Messner, 1991.

Henry, Elizabeth. "Rita Levi-Montalcini, 1909– ," in *Notable Twentieth-Century Scientists*, edited by Emily J. McMurray, Vol. I, pp. 281–283. New York: Gale Research, Inc., 1995.

Holloway, Marguerite. "Finding the Good in the Bad, Profile: Rita Levi-Montalcini." *Scientific American*, Vol. 268, January 1993, pp. 32, 36.

Levi-Montalcini, Rita. *In Praise of Imperfection: My Life and Work*, translated by Luigi Attardi. New York: Basic Books, Inc., 1988.

Liversidge, Anthony. "Interview with Rita Levi-Montalcini." *Omni*, March, 1988, p. 70.

McGrayne, Sharon Bertsch. *Nobel Prize Women in Science*. New York: Birch Lane Press, 1993.

Marx, Jean L. "The 1986 Nobel Prize for Physiology or Medicine." *Science*, October 31, 1986, p. 543.

Pascoe, Elaine. "The 1986 Nobel Prize: Physiology or Medicine." *Grolier's Science Annual*, 1988.

Randall, Frederika. "The Heart and Mind of a Genius." *Vogue*, March 1987, p. 480.

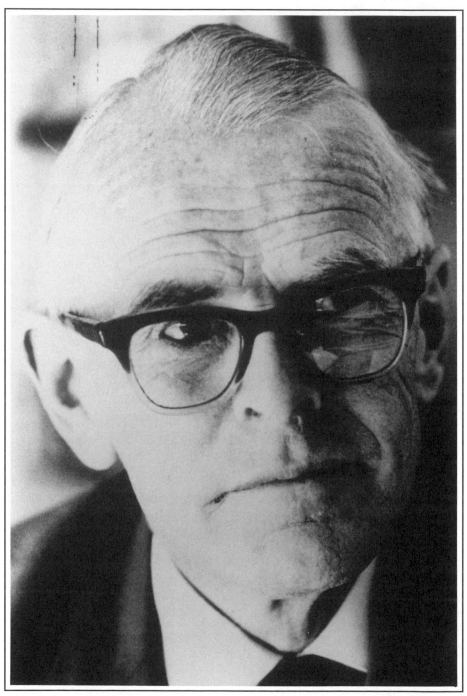

Denis Parsons Burkitt (Courtesy of the National Library of Medicine, Bethesda)

Denis Parsons Burkitt

THE GEOGRAPHIC PATTERNS
OF DISEASE (1911–1993)

W ednesday, 11 October (8:20 P.M.)
We left Kigoma at 8:45 this morning. I have never
traveled through such endless, monotonous African
bush as we did today. Mile after mile, 10 mile after 10
mile, and hundred mile after hundred mile, for 250 miles
on dusty earth roads. Everywhere was dry as dust,
brown and burnt. Just occasionally we went down an
escarpment or through a pass bordered by great rocks.
On the first 60 miles to a Roman Catholic mission we
passed only one car. For the next 170 miles we didn't
pass a single moving vehicle—just three stationary ones.
We saw hardly a soul.
  —from Denis Burkitt's diary on the "Long Safari,"
1961

Uganda is a country of about 20 million people. It covers
an area a little smaller than the state of Oregon, snug
between two big lakes, Mobuto Lake (Lake Albert) and
Victoria Nyanza (Lake Victoria), nestled between Tan-
zania to the east and Zaire to the west. Beginning in
1894, Britain held a protectorate over this country.
When Denis Burkitt arrived in 1961, Uganda was on
the brink of independence, which it gained in 1962.
Burkitt was an Irish physician serving in the Colonial

Service, but for him the position bore no political significance. He was just looking for ways to meet the vast medical challenges faced by the people of this small, hot, rainy country—challenges common to all countries in the tropics. Burkitt's unique gift was that he was able to discern some patterns in these challenges that no one had ever observed before.

Burkitt had no special training beyond his medical school education and a natural ability to perceive patterns in diseases and derive a single hypothesis to explain apparently unconnected data. French epidemiologist Guy de Thé, a long-time friend and colleague, once stated admiringly, "Burkitt is not a scientist; he has no degree, he is just a surgeon, and a military surgeon, which for a Frenchman means he's low grade." De Thé meant this as a compliment, a tribute to Burkitt's innate insights—that a man without the usual academic pedigree could have done so much in understanding the unique diseases affecting Africans.

Denis Burkitt was born in Enniskillen, Northern Ireland, on February 28, 1911, son of James Burkitt, an engineer road-builder who also made his mark in the field of ornithology. Denis was never considered the front runner in his family. He received poor grades in school, and his brother, Robin, was always more popular and better at sports. Denis's loss of an eye in an accident when he was 11 didn't help his grades or sports prowess, yet despite all obstacles, he was determined to be a surgeon. He attended Dublin University, where he obtained his B.A. in 1933 and his M.B. in 1935. He did two years of surgical training and in 1938 became a fellow of Edinburgh's Royal College of Surgeons. Burkitt then served a brief stint as ship's surgeon aboard a freighter between Britain and Manchuria, returning shortly for further surgical training in Plymouth, England, where he met his future wife, Olive Rogers, a student nurse. On completion of his training, Burkitt applied to join the Colonial Medical Service in West Africa, where a friend from college was working. The Colonial Service turned him down because of his missing eye so Burkitt joined the Royal Army Medical Corps, where he served from 1941 to 1946—some of that time, to his delight, in East Africa. He was haunted by the area's beauty and plagued by the need for good medical services there. He resolved to return.

His military duty completed, Burkitt applied again to the Colonial Service, this time with experience on his side, and he succeeded in obtaining an appointment. In 1946 he set out for his first assignment at a rural hospital with only 100 beds, located in Lira, Uganda. Here, he was supposed to serve 200,000 people, with the nearest x-ray machine—and the nearest medical consultant—275 miles away. It was an exercise in self-reliance. Nineteen months later, he received another appointment, to the Makerere University Medical School and Mulago Hospital in Kampala (now the capital city of Uganda).

For centuries, Europeans thought that Africans were cancer-free; cancer appeared to be a uniquely Western disease. But as disease-fighters gained ground over some of the other diseases that plagued the people of this vast continent, the truth became clear: A combination of factors—particularly infections causing diarrhea, malaria, and malnutrition—caused people to die prematurely so that they never reached an

"Burkitt is not a scientist; he has no degree, he is just a surgeon . . . a military surgeon . . ."

—Guy de Thé, French epidemiologist

age when cancer could develop as it did in other populations. However, one morning in 1957, the physician in charge of the pediatric ward at Mulago Hospital called Burkitt in for consultation about a five-year-old boy. The boy's face was "massively swollen, with bizarre lesions involving both sides of his upper and lower jaws." The disease had progressed so far that the child's teeth were loose and his features had become greatly distorted.

Burkitt discounted the idea that the cause might be an infection—not, he thought, in all four quadrants. For the same reason he thought neoplasia (abnormal new tissue) was unlikely. The biopsy results had seemed to indicate some form of granuloma (a mass of inflamed granulation tissue, usually associated with ulcerated infections). Burkitt was stumped. He tried surgery, but neither he nor the referring doctor succeeded in saving the child.

A few weeks later, Burkitt was doing rounds at a hospital on the shore of Victoria Nyanza, about 50 miles away, when he noticed another child, a little girl, with a similarly swollen jaw. He went out to see the child, who was sitting on the grass with her mother, and he noticed a striking resemblance in symptoms to the child at Mulago Hospital. "My interest was riveted immediately," he later wrote.

Burkitt persuaded mother and child to come back with him to Kampala for further examination, during which he noticed a large mass in the child's abdomen. Despite his efforts to save this child, once again everything failed. Burkitt was left only with questions. What could the connection be between a lesion on the jaw and an abdominal mass?

He began to examine other children with jaw tumors and went back through medical records at Mulago Hospital. He found that where there were jaw tumors, growths also existed at certain sites—the eye and eye socket, kidneys, adrenal glands, and ovaries. Occasionally, the liver, testicles, and long bones were involved. Doctors examining these patients had assumed that growths in different areas were the result of separate diseases. At the time, physicians thought tumors were specific to the organs they grew in; no one suspected a connection. But now Burkitt began to believe they'd been wrong—these were neoplastic tumors with all four quadrants of the jaw involved. And, furthermore, Burkitt now saw they were all interconnected.

Once Burkitt had characterized this lymphoma, he began to notice an emerging pattern: Nearly all the cases he encountered occurred in children between two and 14 years of age—most often in children around five years old. He recognized this as another sign that these tumors were distinct from other tumors and had an epidemiology all their own. What began to emerge was that he had found a unique form of cancer.

Burkitt enlisted the help of a nearby medical school, where doctors examined slides of the tumors under microscopes. They discovered that the jaw tumors Burkitt had found and those from different parts of the body in the same children were all the same: a lymphoma, or cancer of the lymph system, that had never been classified before. Moreover, of all the children's tumors recorded in the Kampala Cancer Registry, almost half were this type of lymphoma. This could mean, Burkitt reasoned, that nearly half the tumors afflicting children in Africa were this same malignancy, a cancer of one of the white blood cells, the B cell that normally synthesizes antibodies. (This rapidly fatal cancer of the immune system became known as Burkitt's lymphoma.)

So Burkitt turned to historical records in Uganda and found evidence dating back to the early 1900s of jaw tumors of the same description. He found out from a visiting South African doctor that they virtually never occurred in South Africa, about 1,000 miles away. Why? Burkitt wondered. And if he could find 50 years of history of the disease in East Central Africa, how far south did this pattern extend? He wanted to find what he called the "edge" of the area in which the disease occurred.

He applied for grants, which he received—about 25 pounds or around 67 dollars—and used the money to print up leaflets describing the disease and asking other doctors whether they had ever seen it. He collected mailing lists at medical and scientific conferences and sent out his question-naires, plotting the responses on a map behind his desk. He could only track the study part time—his full-time work was being a government surgeon—and the responses came in slowly, "in dribs and drabs," as he later commented, over a three-year period. In all, about 300 to 400 replies were represented by the map on his wall.

But his hunch was right. There was an "edge" to the distribution. Incidence of the tumors extended in a band across tropical Africa, west to east, about 15 degrees above the equator in the north and 15 degrees below the equator in the south. A sort of tail ran down the east coast, curving down to the border of Mozambique and South Africa. The disease seemed to be confined to this portion of Africa, except for a few cases he heard of in New Guinea. All races and tribes in Africa were susceptible, and even though the tumor did not exist in India, it occurred in Indian children living in Africa. Was there some link to climate or topogra-phy? Why were only certain portions of Africa affected? Burkitt had begun to think in terms of environment. He published his first reports of these statistics in 1958, but few virologists paid any attention. The idea of environmental links to cancer was not common at that time.

Burkitt decided to investigate the area of the distribu-tion—the "lymphoma belt"—for himself, and he organized what he called "the long Safari," an expedition with two colleagues, Edward Williams and Clifford Nelson. He was looking for the distribution's "edge," the dividing line be-tween the regions in which the tumors occurred and where

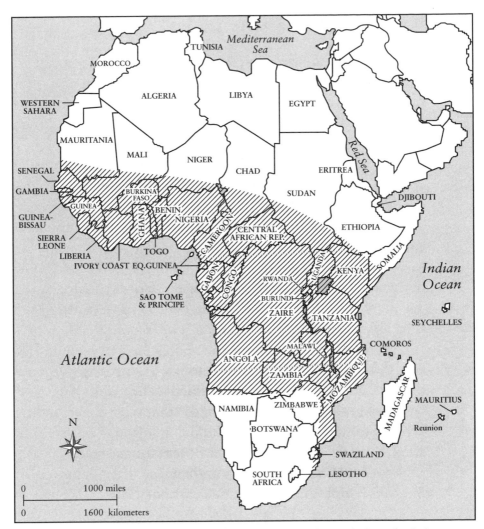

Burkitt's map of Africa in 1962, showing the "lymphoma belt" (shaded area)
(After D. Burkitt)

they didn't. They couldn't hope to cover the whole 5 million square miles of the entire belt, but they mapped out a portion and set out on October 7, 1961, in a battered 1953 Ford station wagon, on a 10,000-mile trip along the eastern portion of Kenya south to the border of South Africa. In ten weeks they covered a distance equal to three times the width of the United States, visiting twelve countries and some sixty hospitals.

They covered every type of terrain, from dry bush to drenched rain forests, from unending flatland to steep mountain passes. They investigated areas of dense population and regions with no one for miles. In his diary, Burkitt described it as "the safari of a lifetime."

Guy de Thé, who later traveled with Burkitt while he worked in Africa and during his travels worldwide working as a viral epidemiologist, once remarked that Burkitt was a stalwart traveler, happily sleeping in muddy tents, robustly eating half-cooked goat and questionable grain mush. He loved the detective work of epidemiology, and his tenacious, determined character probed tirelessly at the evidence. As de Thé remarked about the challenge, "You have to be all the time like a radar, trying to find, to understand."

The results the "safari team" uncovered in hospital records, talking to staff, and examining photos corroborated the data already mapped on Burkitt's office wall. "We suddenly realized," he later recounted, "that we weren't finding an *edge* to the belt. We were finding an *altitude barrier*." In 1962, Burkitt summarized the observations made on this trip, recognizing a correlation between the incidence of Burkitt's lymphoma tumors and location in Africa. He wrote:

> (1) Throughout Uganda, Kenya, and Tanganyika the tumour can occur anywhere except at altitudes of more than about 5000 feet, with the possible exception of the southern part of Tanganyika. (2) The offshore islands of Zanzibar and Pemba are a notable and significant exception. No case of this syndrome has been observed in these islands with a population of more than a quarter of a million. (3) Throughout the Federation of Nyasaland and Southern and Northern Rhodesia [now Zimbabwe], the syndrome is found only in or near the

great river valleys, and on the shores of Lake Nyasa. (4) It is common throughout the coastal plain of Mozambique. (5) It is virtually unknown in South Africa. (6) This pattern of distribution does not coincide with population densities.

What did the areas of the lymphoma belt have in common that others didn't? Burkitt asked. As he looked at a map showing the concentrations of the spread of the disease, a pattern emerged: The cancer occurred with highest frequency where high temperature at low altitude combined with heavy rainfall and abundant water resources. It was exactly the same area as the African malarial belt.

Malaria, long a plague in Africa, is caused by a parasite that is carried by mosquitoes, which breed in stagnant water—and so the disease was most prevalent in Africa in those areas that offered the best conditions for the mosquito to breed in, such as large water sources, heavy rainfall, and warm temperatures at low altitudes. By the 1950s, though, health programs on the islands of Zanzibar and Pemba, off the east coast of Africa, had helped eradicate the mosquitoes' breeding places. These were the same areas that he had noticed were exceptions to the pattern of places that had high rates of Burkitt's lymphoma.

But malaria wasn't the only disease known to be carried by mosquitocs. Researchers had established that mosquitoes transmitted a large group of viruses—now known as the togaviruses—to humans. In fact, the yellow fever virus is one of them. An agent of disease so small it could pass through extremely fine filters, the yellow fever virus was the first such

"We suddenly realized that we weren't finding the *edge* to the belt. We were finding an *altitude barrier.*"

—Denis Parsons Burkitt, recalling the Great Safari

filterable agent to be shown to cause disease in humans.

From all this body of information Burkitt deduced, "The fact that the tumour distribution is dependent on climatic factors strongly suggests that some vector, perhaps a mosquito, is responsible for its transmission. This would naturally suggest that some virus may be the responsible agent."

The association of mosquito-with-virus was a natural step for an epidemiologist to take. But the idea that a mosquito-borne virus could cause or contribute to a cancer was original and caught the imagination of those working with viruses.

In 1961, before leaving on the Long Safari, Burkitt gave a lecture at Middlesex Hospital Medical School in London that attracted the attention of Anthony Epstein (profiled in the next chapter). Upon Burkitt's deduction of the mosquito-born virus, Epstein immediately began an intense hunt for the virus he felt sure was responsible for Burkitt's lymphoma. Others soon followed. Although as early as 1910 Francis Peyton Rous [rhymes with *house*] had associated a virus with tumors in chickens, no one had ever shown a virus to be responsible for tumors in humans. The whole idea seemed strange and, to many, unbelievable. But Anthony Epstein and others picked up where Burkitt left off and proved he was right: Burkitt's lymphoma is caused by a virus.

Strangely, the observation that started the search for a human tumor virus—that a link seemed to exist between mosquito breeding areas and the distribution of the cancer—still remains unexplained. Burkitt developed some ideas on the subject, however, as we'll see in the next chapter.

Burkitt left Africa for England in 1966, but his work with epidemiology was not finished. During the early 1970s, he made still another breakthrough based on his keen ability to observe and draw conclusions from his own experiences—this time by contrasting the diets prevalent in developed and developing countries. As his friend de Thé put it, "Denis has all the qualities of a good observer: He saw a subtle thing and tried to understand it, to pose the right question."

In this case the question he posed was why cancer of the colon was practically nonexistent in Africa. "You know what he did?" de Thé asked in amazement. "Only Denis Burkitt could do it. He weighed the feces! At the end of the twentieth century he weighed the feces!" Burkitt looked at the volume of feces excreted by Africans after eating and calculated the time required for passage and came to the conclusion that the longer material remained in the colon and the smaller the quantity of feces, the greater the chance for colon cancer—and a laundry list of other chronic diseases. It seemed like an archaic approach to his contemporaries—the kind of basic research done by the Italian physician Sanctorius in the 17th century, who weighed himself before and after meals for the better part of 30 years. Burkitt came to the conclusion that people in developed countries would greatly benefit from modifying their diets to include more fiber and less fat and processed carbohydrates.

Since his first pronouncements in the early 1970s, Burkitt's theory about the benefits of dietary fiber has undergone a few twists and turns. Still, no one hypothesis has really explained why colon cancer varies from one population to another. Many medical authorities still recommend fiber-rich diets to promote protection against cancer. In any case, as it turned out, he succeeded in opening up a flood tide of research. As a result, over the following 20 years, new understanding emerged about the role of dietary fiber in general.

In 1992, recognized worldwide as the author of one of the pioneering studies of geographical pathology, Denis Burkitt received the Bower Award in Scientific Achievement at the Franklin Institute in Philadelphia as "the scientist who first linked viruses and cancer and brought fiber into the popular Western diet."

Denis Burkitt died March 23, 1993, of a stroke at his home in Gloucester, England. He was 82. A modest man, he was always passionate about preventing disease and he never ceased searching for patterns that would provide new and better answers.

Chronology

February 28, 1911	Denis Parsons Burkitt born in Enniskillen, Northern Ireland
1933	B.A. degree from Dublin University
1935	M.B. degree from Dublin University
1938	Becomes fellow of Edinburgh's Royal College of Surgeons
1941–46	Serves in the Royal Army Medical Corps
1946	Becomes government surgeon in Uganda
1961	Appointed senior consultant surgeon to the Ugandan Ministry of Health; the Long Safari
1966	The Burkitts leave Africa for London
1970	Publication of *Burkitt's Lymphoma*
1975	Publication of *Refined Carbohydrate Foods and Disease*
1981	Publication of *Western Diseases, Their Emergence and Prevention*
1985	Publication of *Don't Forget Fiber in Your Diet*
1992	Receives Bower Award for linking viruses and cancer in humans and bringing fiber to the popular Western diet
March 23, 1993	Dies in England

Further Reading

Burkitt, Denis P. "The Discovery of Burkitt's Lymphoma." *Cancer* 51, 1983, pp. 1777–1786.

Daintith, John, et al., eds. *Biographical Encyclopedia of Scientists, 2nd Edition*. Vol. 1, p. 132. Bristol: Institute of Physics Publishing, 1994.

Fettner, Anne Guidici. *The Science of Viruses*. New York: Quill/William Morrow, 1990.

Glemsir, B. *Mr. Burkitt and Africa*. New York: The World Publishing Company, 1970.

Radetsky, Peter. *The Invisible Invaders: Viruses and the Scientists Who Pursue Them*. Boston: Little, Brown and Company, 1994.

Trowell, H. C., and D. P. Burkitt, eds. *Western Diseases: Their Emergence and Prevention*. London: Edward Arnold, 1981.

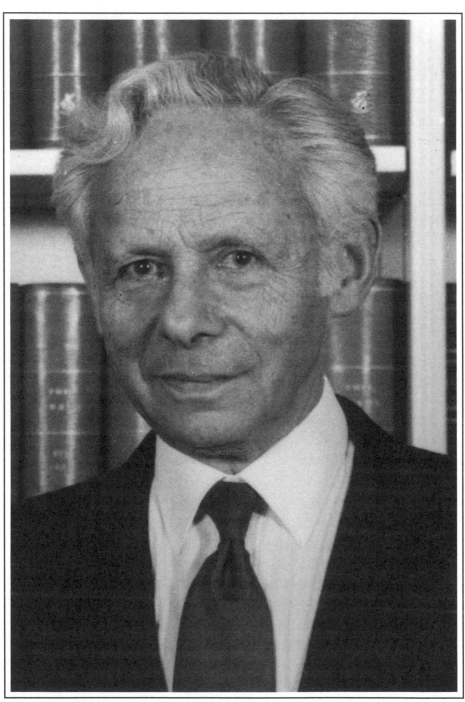

Sir Anthony Epstein in the 1990s (Courtesy of Sir Michael Anthony Epstein)

Sir Michael Anthony Epstein

"AN OBSESSIONAL SORT OF TEMPERAMENT" AND THE EPSTEIN-BARR VIRUS (1921–)

Tony Epstein, a fastidious 40-year-old London researcher at the Middlesex Hospital Medical School, happened to wander by the lecture hall one blustery March day in 1961 and decided to look in. At this unlikely moment, two scientific lives crossed paths and changed Michael Anthony Epstein's entire career. The speaker that day was a rumpled, unsophisticated Irish man with no extensive academic background. He modestly referred to himself as a "bush surgeon," and he was full of tales of his work in Africa. To Epstein it was at first all familiar ground. "Like most speakers from developing countries," Epstein would later remark, "he would show exaggerated examples of this or that kind of disease," trying to gain professional attention for the extreme manifestations of disease he'd found among people who lived in the tropics, often in great poverty.

But the speaker was Denis Burkitt, who had come to talk about Burkitt's lymphoma, the type of cancer he had discovered while working in Uganda, and suddenly the things he said were buzzing in Tony Epstein's mind.

Michael Anthony Epstein was born May 18, 1921, in London. After completing his medical degree at Cambridge University and Middlesex Hospital Medical School, he served from 1945 to 1947 in the British Royal Army Medical Corps and was placed in charge of wives and families of the soldiers in North India. That's when he learned that the clinical practice of general medicine was not for him. "When I came out of the Army," he later told a reporter, "I decided I would rather be in laboratory-based medicine than in any branch of clinical medicine that I'd come across."

After a short period of training in hospital pathology at the Middlesex Hospital Medical School, in the Bland Sutton Institute, he saw an opportunity to continue on at the Institute with the research they were resuming there, after the interruption caused by World War II. The electron microscope had just come into use, and the Bland Sutton Institute had one. (Using an accelerated electron beam instead of visible light, an electron microscope can magnify up to one million times without losing definition. It is therefore very useful for observing extremely small objects.) This one was crude compared to the more sophisticated instruments that later became available, but Epstein and his colleagues found they could gain a good amount of knowledge by comparing the biological activity they could see using conventional microscopes with what they could see in the electron microscope. "I think it was really the first time that this had been done at all," Epstein later told a reporter. "I was using the electron microscope in the very, very earliest days of its application to biological material, and that was quite exciting."

It was during this period that Burkitt came to lecture in London. As Epstein later recounted, "I don't know why, but I caught sight of the notice of his talk and I just went and listened to him."

Burkitt talked about a new tumor—the one for which he is famous and that carries his name, Burkitt's lymphoma. No one outside Africa had ever described this tumor before. (As we've seen, even within Africa, Burkitt's observations had made big news.) Then Burkitt went on to describe his work on the epidemiology of the tumor, showing the correlation between the incidence of the tumor and the climatic factors of temperature and rainfall.

"I'd been listening to this for 20 minutes," Epstein later recalled, "when I was hopping up and down in my seat, absolutely certain that this had to be a human tumor which must be investigated for a virus causation." This idea was so far from common thought at the time that most people considered it ridiculous. Much smaller than a living cell, a virus is a parasite composed of genetic material covered with a protein shell—and it is usually passed in some way from one infected host to another. Generally, researchers had not seen evidence that people became *infected* with cancer from exposure to such a parasite. But Epstein had an instant conviction that this was the avenue that had to be investigated. He invited Burkitt to tea after the lecture and talked with him about having biopsy samples from his patients in East Africa shipped to Middlesex Hospital Medical School. Suddenly everything else Epstein had been working on paled in comparison.

The British Empire Cancer Campaign, later renamed the Cancer Research Campaign, offered financing and arranged to send Epstein to visit Burkitt in his laboratory in Kampala, Uganda. There he made arrangements for overnight air delivery of

"I was hopping up and down in my seat, absolutely certain that this had to be a human tumor which must be investigated for a virus causation."

—Anthony Epstein

biopsy samples. So by the time the rest of the world began to realize the full impact of Burkitt's research, after he reported the results from his epidemiological study, Epstein had already been working for a year on the search for a viral cause. But, even though Epstein had the jump on everyone else, he couldn't create a tissue culture and he couldn't find the virus.

"For two years we tried to get these things to grow," Epstein later remarked. "I tried twenty-four different samples, without success. Obviously, we were doing the wrong things in all our efforts." By this time he'd been joined in the search by another young researcher, Yvonne M. Barr. They tried the standard methods. Nothing. They tried looking through the electron microscope. Still nothing. Morale at the lab sunk lower and lower. With no permanent position at the Institute—in those days few people had that kind of security—and no results to report to the Cancer Research Campaign, which was funding the research, spirits sank to an all-time low. But the track still seemed right to Epstein.

Two years blended into three. Day after day Epstein came to the lab and waited for specimens to arrive from Uganda, hoping that fog wouldn't delay the plane or send it off to Manchester on a three- or four-day detour that would destroy the living tissue. Hoping that the samples would be free of contamination.

Day after day, he and Barr tried to get the tissue samples to grow in a culture so they could investigate further. But they couldn't get the samples to grow, and they couldn't find any trace of a virus. Still, they kept on the problem. They changed the technique, changed the growth medium. Nothing seemed to help. They tried to grow the virus in clots of plasma, as little lumps on grids in a fluid medium, even on tea-bag paper. They also tried to extract the virus to see if they could obtain results by injecting it into mice or developing eggs. Everything failed.

But they kept doggedly on. "It had to be right," Epstein later explained. "It just had the feel of being right. And that's why we carried on."

One Friday the plane was waylaid again, and the shipment reached the lab late in the afternoon, just as everyone was getting ready to leave for the weekend. Epstein and Barr opened the package and looked skeptically at the fluid. It was cloudy—usually a sign that the sample was contaminated with bacteria. Ordinarily they would just throw it out and wait for the next batch. But for some reason, Epstein hesitated.

"I don't know why, but I just didn't want to throw it away." Instead, he took a quick look at the cloudy, unpromising fluid under the microscope. What he saw amazed him. The cloudiness was caused, not by bacteria, but by huge numbers of single cells floating in the fluid. This reminded Epstein of a technique he'd seen on a visit to the Yale University School of Medicine, so he broke the tumor material up into a suspension of single cells and then tried to grow the tumor in tissue culture. That, at last, was productive—it was the first time anyone had ever succeeded in growing human lymphocytes in a continuous culture.

But the virus they had set out to look for still eluded them. Epstein, Barr and now another assistant, B. G. Achong, tried every method they could think of—all the standard techniques for isolating a virus. Every test came up negative. But now, with the new cultured material they had developed, they were able to section it at last and take a look under the electron microscope. So every time they ran a biological test, Epstein would double-check the results, to see what he could see, under the electron microscope as well.

"There, in the very first grid square was the cell with unequivocal virus particles. There was no doubt whatsoever," he later declared. Shaken, Epstein turned off the electron microscope, fearful that the heat of the machine would damage the specimen. It was there. It really was there. Calmly, he went for a walk around the block. Then he circled the block once, twice more. All the while he was thinking. This was it. He was sure.

In 1964, Michael Anthony Epstein joined with his colleagues, B. G. Achong and Yvonne M. Barr to describe the Epstein-Barr virus (EBV) for the first time in a paper they published in the journal *Science*. But, while the battle was won, the war was not over yet. "We were able to identify the *kind* of virus, but not exactly what it was," Epstein later explained. "That is, we knew the family: it was one of the herpes group. But it wasn't any *known member* of the herpes group."

Furthermore, fellow researchers weren't ready to believe it. Unaccustomed to the use of the electron microscope, they referred to the particles as "virus-like" particles. The EBV didn't behave the way they expected it to, and no one in Britain would touch it. Finally, Epstein and Barr found a team of researchers at the Children's Hospital in Philadelphia—Werner and Gertrude Henle [HEN lee]—who were willing to collaborate with them. The Henles showed that antibodies existed in the blood of Burkitt's patients. They also showed that these antibodies reacted with antigens that existed within the tumor tissues.

> "There, in the very first grid square was the cell with unequivocal virus particles."
>
> —Anthony Epstein

We now know that the Epstein-Barr virus is a virus that does demonstrate biological activity, but it's a special kind of activity that no one knew how to look for then. That's why ordinary tests for the presence of a virus hadn't worked. Not until the electron microscope showed it in a new way did the truth begin to emerge. Epstein and Achong showed in a paper, published in 1979, that EBV is a unique herpes virus.

Researchers have since shown that the Epstein-Barr virus has worldwide distribution, and the Henles showed its association with mononucleosis—sometimes known as the "kissing disease" because it is transmitted primarily in saliva. Most people, as it turns out, carry the virus from early childhood.

This evidence pretty much cast aside Burkitt's original idea that Burkitt's lymphoma was transmitted by insects. Burkitt retracted his hypothesis, commenting, "I have on many occasions publicly stated my conviction that no progress is made in medical research—or in happy marriage—unless mistakes are openly admitted."

So then, why does Burkitt's lymphoma occur only in some restricted areas? Epstein and Burkitt argued that only in cases in which malaria or some other chronic condition has suppressed a child's immature immune system, could the virus provoke lymphoid cells into malignant growth—and that's why Burkitt's lymphoma occurs in the same areas as malaria. In industrial countries where malaria is not so widespread, the virus doesn't turn up until later years, when it causes mononucleosis, generally a less serious disease.

Some studies have also suggested an association of EBV with other cancers, as well as AIDS. And in recent years it has been connected with Epstein-Barr syndrome, or chronic fatigue syndrome, a disease that occurs typically among financially comfortable individuals in executive or middle-management positions in industrial nations. How the same virus could cause such a diversity of diseases in so many different scenarios remains a mystery, but studies do show a high incidence of the virus or its antibodies in blood tests.

The EBV saga remains an evolving story and not all its significance is yet known. But the story of its discovery demonstrates the essence of science at work.

What is the essence of science to Tony Epstein? "There are different ways of doing things," he once said, "and I think that certain kinds of meticulousness and fussing over details are important and should be passed on to younger people." This focus on minutiae, he emphasized, was essential to the scientific process—a process that he believes derives from "an obsessional sort of temperament." For him an unflinching, persistent hands-on approach has paid off. "You've got to keep messing about at the bench," he says. "You see how to change this just a little bit, and you see how to change that a bit, and you want to tinker with something and find a slightly different and new way of doing it. You make a little bit of apparatus . . ." Finally, you just may find something.

And that is likely to be just the beginning.

It was for Michael Anthony Epstein, whose work has received international recognition, including the Paul Ehrlich and Ludwig Darmstaedter Prize and Medal (West Germany, 1973), Bristol Myers Award for Cancer Research (United States, 1982), Prix Griffuel (France, 1986), Gairdner International Award (Canada, 1988), and the Royal Medal from the Royal Society of London (1992). He was elected a fellow of the Royal Society of London in 1979 and was knighted in 1991.

Chronology

May 18, 1921	Michael Anthony Epstein born in London
1945–47	Serves in Royal Army Medical Corps
1947	Returns to Middlesex Hospital as assistant pathologist
1956	Epstein travels to the United States, where he learns electron microscope techniques
1961	Epstein hears Denis Burkitt speak in London

1964	M. Anthony Epstein, B. G. Achong, and Yvonne M. Barr announce their discovery of a herpes virus-like particle in Burkitt's lymphoma cells
1965	Becomes professor of pathology at Bristol University
1985	Retires from Bristol, but continues his work in the Department of Clinical Medicine at Oxford
1991	Epstein is knighted

Further Reading

Daintith, John, et al., eds. *Biographical Encyclopedia of Scientists, 2nd Edition.* Vol. 1, p. 265. Bristol: Institute of Physics Publishing, 1994.

Epstein, M. A., B. G. Achong, and Y. M. Barr. "Virus particles in cultured lymphoblasts from Burkitt's lymphoma." *Lancet* 1, 1964, pp. 702–703.

Epstein, M. A., and B. G. Achong. *The Epstein-Barr Virus.* New York: Springer-Verlag, 1979.

Fettner, Ann Giudici. *The Science of Viruses.* New York: Quill, an imprint of William Morrow and Co., 1990, pp. 117–124.

Levine, Arnold J. *Viruses.* New York: Scientific American Library, 1992, pp. 76–85.

Radetsky, Peter. *The Invisible Invaders: Viruses and the Scientists Who Pursue Them.* Boston: Little, Brown and Company, 1994, pp. 173–193.

Wolpert, Lewis, and Alison Richards. "Between the Lines," interview with Anthony Epstein in *A Passion for Science.* Oxford: Oxford University Press, 1988.

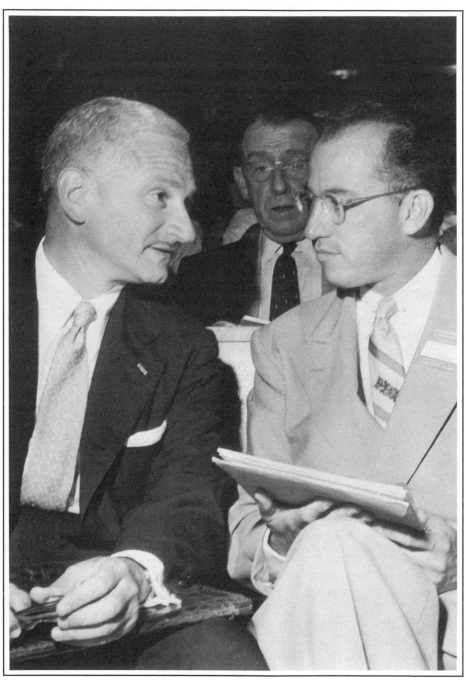

Albert Bruce Sabin (left) and Jonas Salk together at a conference in Italy (Courtesy of the University of Cincinnati)

Jonas Salk and Albert Bruce Sabin

(1914–1995)   (1906–1993)

PREVENTING POLIO

E verything was going well for Franklin Delano Roosevelt in August 1921. He was a wealthy young man with a law practice in New York, a future in politics, and a vacation stretching before him. As usual, he was spending the summer with his family on Campobello Island in New Brunswick, Canada. On August 10, they'd just headed back from a day of sailing, when Roosevelt spotted a forest fire burning out of control on a nearby island. He and his sons raced to shore to help beat back the fire. That night, exhausted and chilled, he returned to the cottage and went to bed early. But the next day something was wrong. Usually athletic and fit, when he got up, one leg dragged strangely and wouldn't take his weight. His temperature soared to 102 degrees, with pain in his back and legs. Franklin Roosevelt had come down with polio, and he would never walk on his own again.

For most people growing up in the 1950s, Jonas Salk and Albert Sabin were giant-killers. But the giant they slayed was actually so tiny that even the finest filters didn't catch it and ordinary microscopes couldn't detect it. Yet it raged through the United States during the first half of the 20th century, leaving thousands of children paralyzed for life, or dead, and causing panic and fear in the hearts of thousands of others.

Infantile paralysis, or poliomyelitis as it is more often called now, is a very old disease. Paintings and drawings that depict people with withered legs suggest that the disease existed at least as long ago as ancient Egypt. Firm documentation from the 19th century tells us that a few small epidemics occurred in the 1880s. But no serious epidemics occurred until the 20th century—most likely because polio is a "disease of civilization." Because it is spread through fecal matter, most children in areas with low sanitation standards obtain an early immunity to it—much as children in undeveloped countries become immune early to diseases like mononucleosis, caused by the Epstein-Barr virus. Improvements in sanitation remove this early exposure to the polio virus and immunity doesn't build up, so when older children under these conditions are exposed to the polio virus, they have no resistance.

Polio epidemics occurred throughout the world in the early 20th century, in all the major cities of Europe, Australia and elsewhere. But the United States was hit especially hard. In New York City alone, 9,000 cases occurred in 1916, with 27,000 across the nation. Panic set in. People fled from the cities in the summer, when the epidemics seemed to hit. They began to talk of quarantines and the cholera epidemic of the 1890s. For the next four decades, fear arrived every summer. Children were kept out of public pools and public fountains were off limits. People were frightened. They wanted someone to do something about it.

Franklin Roosevelt was partly responsible for the successful campaign against polio. He put his name behind it. He supported the establishment of a rehabilitation center at Warm Springs, Georgia (more a nice idea than an effective one). And he encouraged people to give to the March of Dimes campaign launched by the National Foundation for

Infantile Paralysis, probably the most successful campaign in the history of charity drives.

The man who ran that campaign, Basil O'Connor, was also the funding power behind the development of both successful vaccines—the killed virus vaccine developed by Jonas Salk and the attenuated live virus vaccine developed by Albert Sabin. (O'Connor can be seen looking over the shoulders of the two researchers in the photograph at the beginning of this chapter.)

The American public had come to have high expectations of biomedical research in the early part of the century, and by the 1930s and 1940s it was widely anticipated that science would find a way to prevent polio. The virus that caused this disease that crippled and killed the young had already been found (research in the 1930s had distinguished several types of polio virus); the factors that caused its spread had become understood; and the pathology of the disease had been established. Now the race was on to develop a vaccine.

JONAS EDWARD SALK

Jonas Edward Salk was born October 28, 1914, in East Harlem, New York. He was the oldest son of Daniel B. Salk, a garment worker who enjoyed sketching, and Dora Press. His parents, who came from an Orthodox Jewish heritage in Poland, encouraged their son's academic abilities. A highly motivated achiever, Salk attended Townsend Harris High School for the gifted, graduating at 15. He immediately entered City College of New York to study law, but became intrigued by his science courses. He earned his bachelor's degree in science at 19 and, using money borrowed by his parents, he entered the New York University School of

Medicine. The year was 1933, and Franklin Roosevelt had just been elected president of the United States. Money was scarce for everyone because of the Great Depression that lasted throughout most of the 1930s. But after his first year in medical school, Salk's scholastic record earned him scholarships and fellowships that paid his tuition. During his last year in medical school he met Thomas Francis, Jr., who would become a key collaborator on the most important work of his career.

On June 27, 1939, Salk received his M.D. degree, and the next day he married Donna Lindsay, a social worker with a Phi Beta Kappa key and a degree in psychology. After graduation, Salk began a two-year internship at the Mount Sinai Hospital in New York. As he was completing the internship at Mount Sinai, Salk received an invitation from Francis to join him at the University of Michigan, where Francis headed the department of epidemiology. It was a difficult move for two native New Yorkers, but the Salks decided they couldn't pass up the opportunity. There, under a grant from the U.S. Army, Salk and Francis began working on the development of an influenza vaccine. In 1918, during World War I, the most destructive epidemic of modern times, an influenza outbreak—made worse by wartime conditions—had caused an estimated 20 million deaths. Now with World War II in full force, troops all over the world were again side by side in the trenches.

What Salk and Francis were trying to create was a substance that would cause the body to make antibodies without producing any sign of illness. They were working with "killed-virus" vaccines, composed of killed flu viruses that would trigger the body's immune system. Using formalin to kill the viruses, by 1943 Francis and Salk had developed a vaccine effective against both prevalent types of flu, A and B. They began clinical trials, the first stage of putting the vaccine to work, giving shots to a group of people under carefully controlled conditions.

In 1946, Salk became assistant professor of epidemiology at the University of Michigan. However, hoping to gain more control over his research, he accepted a position the following year at the University of Pittsburgh's School of Medicine's Virus Research Laboratory as assistant professor of bacteriology. The move, though, did not initially look promising. The lab was not up to par, and the technicians had no experience with the kind of basic research he'd been doing. Salk worked aggressively getting funding for the expansion of laboratory facilities and soon had the Pittsburgh lab prepared for cutting-edge viral research.

By this time, scientific papers by Salk had gained the attention of O'Connor, the director of the National Foundation for Infantile Paralysis. They met, and O'Connor convinced Salk to work on the polio vaccine that the foundation wanted to sponsor. O'Connor was so impressed with Salk that he decided to invest nearly all the Foundation's research money in the Salk polio vaccine effort—a questionable decision, but one he had the power to make.

A great deal of groundwork was already being laid in polio research when Salk came on the scene. At Children's Hospital in Boston, John Enders, Thomas Weller, and Frederick Robbins had been working on growing the polio virus in culture, and by 1949, they had successfully grown the polio virus in several types of human and animal tissue. Until then, Salk and most other researchers had thought only nerve tissue could be used, since, at that time, polio was thought to be a disease of the nervous system.

But in 1952, another team of researchers established the virus's course of entry: through the digestive tract, where it resided in the bloodstream for a time, and then on to the tissues of the nervous system in the brain and spine. Once there, it launched a full attack on the body. This was important news because it meant a counterattack could be fought against the virus in the bloodstream.

By now Salk was working for the foundation and receiving reports from all the other researchers working on polio. The flow of information from other laboratories and scientists made a new level of focus and clarity possible. Salk now knew where the polio virus entered the body, how it grew, when it attacked, and how to grow his own cultures of the virus in his lab. Now the problem was to develop a vaccine safe for human use.

Although other laboratories were investigating attenuated- or weakened-virus vaccines, Salk believed that the only safe vaccine was one composed of dead viruses—a very controversial position. Proponents of the attenuated virus felt that a dead virus would not cause the body to produce enough antibodies to provide effective protection. But Salk stuck with his theory—that the only safe virus is a dead virus—and began looking for the exact strength of formaldehyde needed to do the job. If he used too little, not all the viruses would die, and the vaccine might cause polio in vaccinated patients. If he used too much, he might weaken the effective power of the vaccine.

He tested his formulas systematically on monkeys. By this time he had also shown that all known strains of polio virus fall into three groups. So he repeated the test for each of the three strains. First he would kill the virus with a carefully measured dosage, letting it sit in the formaldehyde for 13 days. (He could detect no sign of life after three days, but he wanted to leave a wide margin for error, which he calculated at one trillion to one.) Then he would inject a well monkey. If the monkey contracted the disease, he would know the formaldehyde wasn't strong enough and he would begin again. Lives depended on the results, so he exhaustively repeated his experiments.

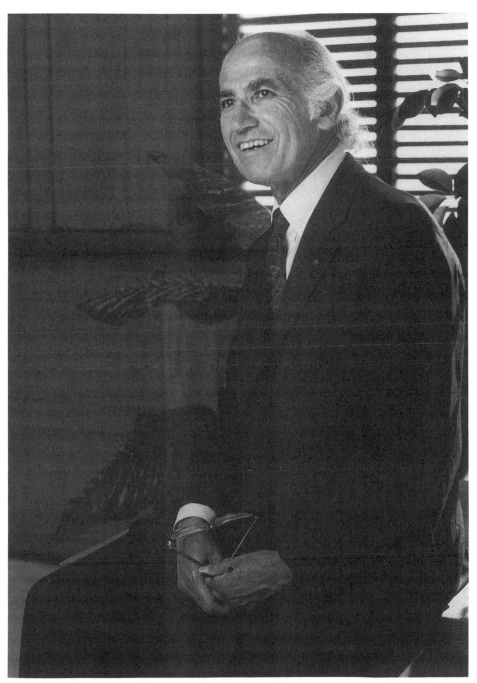

As head of the Salk Institute, Salk continued his search for ways to defeat disease (Courtesy of the Salk Institute)

By 1952, he thought he had produced a vaccine that would be reasonably effective against all three strains of polio. But researchers who had been in the field of polio research longer than he remained skeptical. Among them, Albert Sabin was the chief proponent of the live-virus vaccine.

But Salk proceeded. First, in a preliminary trial, he gave the vaccine to children who had already been infected with the polio virus. Since they were already immune, if it didn't work, they still wouldn't contract polio. But their immune systems should boost the number of antibodies if the vaccine was working. It worked. The vaccine pushed the antibodies significantly higher.

Salk announced the development of the vaccine at the beginning of 1953, which probably was a mistake. He said his intention was only to provide hope. But other scientists were dismayed at his lack of scientific protocol, which calls for due process in publishing results: Get all your facts, and then publish. They felt he was grandstanding.

But Salk was sure that the vaccine was ready for massive field trials. In the largest medical experiment ever run in the United States, he began preparations to inoculate over 400,000 children. Finally the preparations were finished and the trials began in April 1954. Thomas Francis directed the trials, which were sponsored by the National Infantile Paralysis Society. As it turned out, over a million children between the ages of six and nine were inoculated during this trial stage. One-third received three injections, one for each type of polio virus, plus one booster shot. A second third

"What had the most profound effect was the freedom from fear."

—Jonas Salk, in 1995, looking back 40 years after the official announcement of the Salk vaccine received a placebo shot. And a final group received nothing.

Finally, all the results were in, and on April 12, 1955, it was official—Jonas Salk's vaccine was pronounced effective, potent, and safe in nearly 90 percent of the cases. Five hundred of the world's top scientists and doctors attended the announcement, as well as 150 journalists and 16 TV and movie crews. The uproar was enormous. Salk was a hero.

Unfortunately for Salk, who wanted out of the limelight by this time, a tragic accident happened. Salk had personally taught his procedure for killing the virus and preparing the vaccine to personnel at all the manufacturing sites, which were private-sector pharmaceutical manufacturing firms. But just two weeks after the announcements, one of the manufacturers made an error. Nearly 200 children injected with certain lots of the Salk vaccine came down with paralytic poliomyelitis and 11 died. For a time it looked like the entire vaccine program would have to be abandoned. But all the problem vaccines were traced to one manufacturer, Cutter Laboratories of California. On May 7 the surgeon general called a halt to the vaccine program. An investigation showed Cutter had used faulty batches of a virus that was resistant to the formaldehyde. New safeguards and standards were enacted, and the program resumed.

By the summer of 1955, over 5 million children had received polio shots. Over the next two years, more than 200 million doses of Salk vaccine were given. And not one further incidence of paralysis resulted from any of the vaccine.

By the summer of 1961, the number of polio cases had dropped 96 percent compared to the previous 5 years. The polio epidemic was over at last.

After continuing work in preventative and experimental medicine at Pittsburgh, Jonas Salk founded the Salk Institute for Biological Studies in La Jolla, California, in 1960. Since then the Institute's cutting-edge biological research facilities have attracted many highly qualified researchers from all over the world. When the new Institute opened in 1963, Salk continued to devote himself to new challenges, including the study of multiple sclerosis, cancer, and AIDS.

He once again achieved a degree of notoriety when he married Françoise Gilot, the former wife of Pablo Picasso, two years after divorcing Donna.

Salk is the author of several books on the philosophy of science, which he wrote in the 1970s. In 1977 he received the Presidential Medal of Freedom, and in 1995, Salk jubilantly celebrated the 40th anniversary of his successful development of the polio vaccine.

In the early 1990s, many people hoped Salk might find a vaccine against the HIV virus, which causes AIDS, but in 1993, he reported that the experimental AIDS vaccine developed by his research team had not shown good results, neither slowing the course of the disease nor decreasing its severity. Salk, however, seemed to take such disappointments in stride. The man who had personally done much of the work to perform the exacting, repetitive tests required to develop a safe polio vaccine in the 1950s was not one to get discouraged easily.

As he said to one journalist, "To a scientist, fame is neither an end nor even a means to an end. Do you recall what Emerson said?—'The reward of a thing well done is the opportunity to do more.'" Jonas Salk died on June 24, 1995.

> "Wisdom, understood as a new kind of strength, is a paramount necessity for man. Now, even more than ever before, it is required as a basis for fitness, to maintain life itself on the face of this planet, and as an alternative to paths toward alienation and despair."
>
> —Jonas Salk, 1973, in his book *The Survival of the Wisest*

ALBERT BRUCE SABIN

Born August 26, 1906, in Belostok, Russia (now Bialystok, Poland), Albert Bruce Sabin was 15 when he left Russia for the United States with his parents, Jacob and Tillie Sabin. His family had sought to escape the extreme poverty of czarist Russia. They settled in Paterson, New Jersey, and Sabin's father pursued the silk and textile business. After graduation from Paterson High School in 1923, Sabin needed to settle on a career, and an uncle volunteered to pay for his college education if Sabin would study dentistry. So Sabin set out for New York University dental school, but during the next two years, he came across a book called *The Microbe Hunters* by Paul deKruif, and became fascinated by virology. (The heroic and romantic vision of the same book would also influence Gertrude Elion.) So Sabin dropped out of dental school in favor of medicine. Now no longer supported by his uncle, he worked his way through school with odd jobs and scholarships. In 1931 he received his M.D. degree from New York University and completed his residency in pathology, surgery, and internal medicine at Bellevue Hospital in New York City.

Very early in his career, while still in residency, Sabin began to show his talent as a viral researcher. In 1932 he isolated the B virus from a colleague who had died after a monkey had bitten him. He soon was able to establish that the B virus's natural habitat was the monkey. He also showed that it was related to the human herpes simplex virus.

After doing research at the Lister Institute of Preventive Medicine in London, Sabin worked at the Rockefeller Institute for Medical Research in New York in 1935. Later, in 1939, he joined the staff of the Children's Hospital Research Foundation and the College of Medicine of the University of Cincinnati, where he spent the rest of his career.

Beginning as early as 1931, Sabin spent many years in search of protective vaccines against the strains of polio viruses that had been discovered. His approach, though, was completely different from Jonas Salk's. Sabin was looking for a polio strain that could be used in live, attenuated form.

Although Salk's announcement of the dead-virus vaccine seemed to have won the race in 1953, the accident with the Cutter Laboratories vaccine caused Sabin to renew his efforts. Sabin had warned that a dead-virus vaccine could actually be more dangerous than the attenuated-virus approach. And the accident seemed to lend support to his point of view.

Sabin's idea was to work toward a vaccine that could be orally administered. Then the virus would multiply in the intestinal tract instead of being injected directly into the bloodstream. He performed meticulous tests on monkeys to see if the diluted viruses he was using were sufficiently weakened so they wouldn't damage the nervous system. He performed experiments on 9,000 to 15,000 monkeys over the course of his testing.

"Unless you set yourself a definite target for completing work in a certain field, you can go on asking yourself questions forever."

—Albert Sabin in 1960

Once he had the vaccine, he tested it on himself and his family. Prisoners from the Chillicothe Prison in Ohio also volunteered. The vaccine was safe. It produced immunity with no negative side effects. But Sabin could not obtain backing for large-scale trials in the United States. However, he did convince the Health Ministry in the Soviet Union to run massive trials using his vaccine. The World Health Organization in Geneva also supported Sabin's effort, believing that it would have a more successful worldwide effect than Salk's vaccine. Rus-

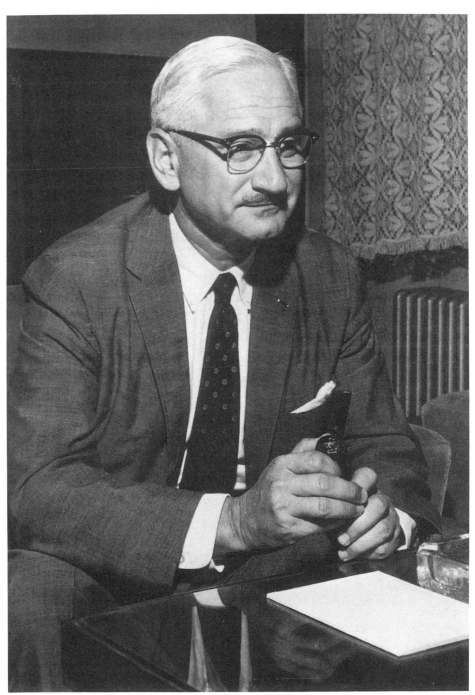

Albert Sabin (Courtesy of the University of Cincinnati)

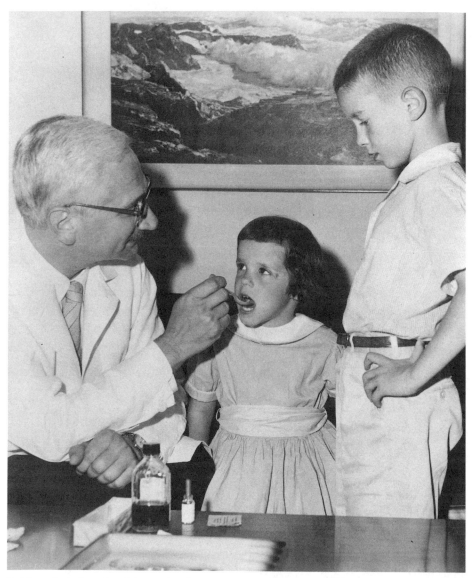

Sabin administering his oral polio vaccine   (Courtesy of the University of Cincinnati)

sian children began receiving the vaccine in 1957, and millions received the vaccine over the next few years.

Finally, in 1960, the U.S. Public Health Service approved the Sabin vaccine to be manufactured in the United States. After that breakthrough, the oral vaccine, which is far easier to administer, virtually took over in the United States as well as worldwide. Sabin remained active in research well into his seventies, traveling in 1980 to Brazil to help eradicate a new outbreak of polio there. He also researched the role of viruses in cancer.

The controversy between the two researchers continued, however, when Salk wrote an opinion editorial published in the *New York Times* in 1973, urging people to return to his vaccine to avoid the risks he said the Sabin vaccine posed. Years later in 1990, Sabin summed up his rival's work with the pithy comment, "It was pure kitchen chemistry. Salk didn't discover anything." The two men remained opposed until Sabin's death, March 3, 1993. At that time Salk issued a statement praising Sabin's work in the fight against polio.

When people are racing, they tend to cut corners, and the race to produce a polio vaccine was no exception. In some ways, both Salk and Sabin came out winners. Salk got there first, but Sabin's vaccine was easier to administer, and so it replaced the Salk vaccine. Yet few people remember Sabin's name. Dozens of books line library shelves detailing the adventure of the Salk vaccine; but Sabin, oddly, remains almost forgotten.

There was nothing rosy about the way the race was run, either: premature announcements raised false hopes, trial testing was mishandled, disasters occurred in early vaccine testing, and Sabin and Salk showed less than professional restraint in their rivalry. But none of this changes the results.

Thanks to Salk and Sabin's polio vaccines, by the 1990s polio rarely occurred among the developed nations. Optimism had grown so greatly

"It was pure kitchen chemistry. Salk didn't discover anything."

—Albert Sabin on Salk's work, 1990

by 1985 that the World Health Organization (WHO) began a worldwide effort to eradicate polio by 2000. No case of polio has been reported in the Americas since 1991.

Chronology—Jonas Salk

October 28, 1914	Jonas Edward Salk is born in New York City
1934	Graduates from City College of New York
1939	Receives medical degree from New York University
1942–47	Immunological work at University of Michigan
1947	Becomes director of viral research laboratory at University of Pittsburgh
1953	Announces development of killed virus polio vaccine
1954	Nationwide trials are begun of Salk's killed-virus vaccine, the first effective killed-virus vaccine against polio
April 1955	Success of the "Salk Vaccine" tests announced
More than 100 cases of paralytic poliomyelitis develop among Americans injected with certain lots of Salk vaccine produced by Cutter Laboratories
1960	Salk founds the Salk Institute for Biological Studies at the University of California at San Diego
1963	Salk becomes director of the Salk Institute
1975	Salk retires as director of the Salk Institute

| 1987 | Begins search for vaccine for AIDS |
| June 24, 1995 | Jonas Salk dies |

Chronology—Albert Bruce Sabin

August 26, 1906	Albert Sabin is born in Belostok, Russia (now Bialystok, Poland)
1921	Sabin arrives in the United States of America
1931	Receives medical degree from New York University
1935	Joins scientific staff at Rockefeller Institute for Medical Research
1939	Begins teaching pediatrics at University of Cincinnati
1957	Develops a live-virus vaccine against polio, which eventually replaces Jonas Salk's killed-virus vaccine
1961	Sabin's oral vaccine is licensed
1969	Leaves Cincinnati to become president of the Weizmann Institute of Science, Israel
March 3, 1993	Sabin dies in Washington, D.C.

Further Reading

Carter, Richard. *Breakthrough: The Saga of Jonas Salk*. New York: Trident Press, 1966.

Fettner, Anne Giudici. *The Science of Viruses*. New York: Quill/William Morrow, 1990.

Radetsky, Peter. *The Invisible Invaders: Viruses and the Scientists Who Pursue Them*. Boston: Little, Brown and Company, 1994.

Rowland, John. *The Polio Man*. New York: Roy Publishers, 1960.

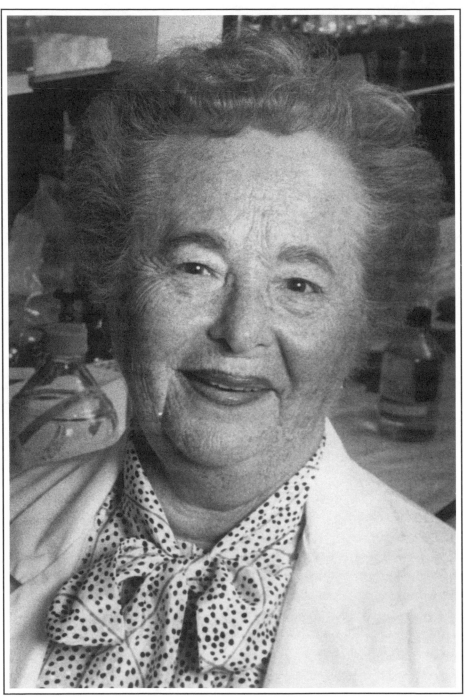

Gertrude Belle Elion (Courtesy of Glaxo Wellcome)

Gertrude Belle Elion

THE "PURINE PATH TO CHEMOTHERAPY" (1918–)

The old man had been a watchmaker in Russia, but when his eyesight had faded 13 years before, he had traveled to New York, where he had relatives. By then retired, he loved to take his little red-haired granddaughter to the park or sit and tell her stories. Like much of his family, he was a biblical scholar, so he knew a lot of stories to keep her interested, and he often told them in Yiddish.

Now he lay dying in a hospital bed, suffering and in pain, and his young granddaughter, only 16, agonized with him as she stood by his bedside. There was nothing she could do to ease the pain or fight the long, slow progress of the stomach cancer from which he would finally die.

For Trudy Elion [ELL ee uhn], that was the moment she decided what she would do with her life. "That was the turning point," she later explained. "It was as though the signal was there: 'This is the disease you're going to have to work against.'"

Gertrude Elion's successful fight against leukemia, gout, herpes, and many other diseases proved to be extraordinary in many ways. It began slowly. The early portion of her resume includes a list of ignoble tasks, including checking vanilla beans for freshness, examining fruit for mold, and checking pickles for acidity. She never finished her Ph.D. She chose chemistry over biology to avoid performing dissections. But she abundantly fulfilled her vow to pursue—and in some cases win—the fight against diseases like the cancer that killed her grandfather. In 1988, she received the Nobel Prize in physiology or medicine, a distinction she shared with her former boss, George H. Hitchings, and with Sir James W. Black of Great Britain. And in 1991 Elion became the first woman ever inducted into the National Inventors' Hall of Fame in Akron, Ohio.

"Trudy" Elion, as her friends call her, was born in 1918, two years before women earned the right to vote in the United States. As Rita Levi-Montalcini also found in Italy, Elion soon discovered that women met with little encouragement in the sciences in those days. Also, unfortunately, Elion emerged from college in 1937, right in the midst of a worldwide economic depression. Jobs and academic financial aid were scarce for everyone, especially women. Although she graduated *summa cum laude* (with highest honors) from New York City's Hunter College, 15 colleges turned down her application for financial aid for graduate studies. She took several marginal laboratory jobs, one without pay, just to gain experience, but she met with opposition. As she later told a reporter, she was told, "We don't have women in the laboratory; you'd be a very distracting influence on the men." She attended New York University part-time to work on her master's degree, which she earned in 1941. And she taught chemistry and physics for a brief time in the New York City high school system. But, despite the obstacles, she remained enthusiastic and determined "to become a great research scientist," as she told one job interviewer. His name was Charles Frey, and years later he could still recall her disappointment when all he could offer her was a job washing out test tubes in a laboratory—for which she was obviously overqualified.

But Elion came from a family of immigrants who were used to using their brains to overcome adversity. Elion's father, Robert Elion, had arrived in New York from Lithuania when he was 12. His family heritage was one of educated achievers—one relative traced the line of rabbis in the family back through historical records as far as the year 700—and young Robert worked nights in a drugstore so he could go to the New York University School of Dentistry. He graduated in 1914 and was successful in his profession and in investments. He loved music—often taking Trudy to the opera—and was known in his community for his wisdom and intelligence.

Her mother, Bertha Cohen, also came from a Jewish Eastern European family with a strong scholarly tradition—Bertha's grandfather had been a high priest. When she was 14 she emigrated from her home in an area of Russia that is now in Poland, sent to live with older sisters in New York. Gentle and practical, Bertha learned English at night school and entered the clothing trade. At the age of 19 she married Robert Elion.

As a child, Trudy Elion loved school. "It didn't matter if it was history, languages, or science. I was just like a sponge." Her favorite heroes were Marie Curie and Louis Pasteur—"people who discovered things." She had a gift for explaining, and she often helped her brother Herbert, six years younger, with his homework. She always took it for granted that she would go to college.

But in 1929, despite the urging of relatives, Robert Elion did not sell his stocks as the market became unstable. Selling out, he reasoned, would add to the panic and hurt other investors. When the crash came in October 1929, he lost everything and spent the rest of his life trying to repay his debts. So, just as Trudy Elion was entering high school, her hopes for a university education became bleak. Her high grades, however, gained her admission to Hunter College, at that time the women's branch of City College of New York, where tuition was free to those who qualified for entrance. The all-female environment, with 75 majoring in chemistry, did not prepare her for the inhospitable job market she faced upon graduation. Most of her chemistry classmates, she later realized, expected to teach, not do research.

Still, Elion never lost her naturally graceful assertiveness. And she never felt she suffered from the lack of female role models in the sciences. As she told a reporter for the *Washington Post*, "I never considered that I was a woman and then a scientist. My role models didn't have to be women—they could be scientists."

Finally, in 1944, she got a break. When men left the work force to serve in the armed services during World War II, jobs in industry and laboratory research began to open up for women. That's when George Hitchings of Wellcome Research Laboratories in Tuckahoe, New York (part of Burroughs Wellcome Company), offered her a position as a researcher working with nucleic acids (RNA and DNA). This was a new field, known to be a key to genetics, even though James Watson and Francis Crick had not yet uncovered the structure of DNA (deoxyribonucleic acid).

Instead of using the sort of trial-and-error method that had often been used in the past to discover new drugs, Hitchings wanted to approach the job from a more rational, scientific knowledge base. He reasoned that all cells require nucleic acids to reproduce, but the rapid growth of certain cells—those found in bacteria, tumors, and protozoa—must require especially large amounts of nucleic acids. Hitchings was working on ways to interfere with nucleic acid metabolism in cells in a way that would defeat the human cells' enemies—by blocking reproduction of bacteria and cancerous tumor cells, as well as viruses—without harming the normal host cells. He divided up the components of the nucleic acids among his staff.

Elion's assignment was to investigate purines, a major group of compounds. As it turned out, it was a very productive assignment, since the purine bases—adenine and guanine—are the building blocks of DNA and RNA (ribonucleic acid). She was fascinated and felt like a pioneer. This was largely unexplored territory, and she spent long hours trying hundreds of experiments to find out what each new piece of microbiological evidence meant.

As she later recalled, "We were exploring new frontiers, since very little was known about nucleic acid biosynthesis or the enzymes involved with it. . . . Each series of studies was like a mystery story in that we were constantly trying to deduce what the microbiological results meant, with little biochemical information to help us."

As head of the laboratory, Hitchings gave her a lot of freedom to pursue all sides of the questions, find out how the chemicals worked; and she pursued thirstily. She was publishing results within two years, and here again, Hitchings encouraged her to write her own papers and list her name first, as the first researcher in the work. Eventually she published more than 225 papers, and soon became part of the academic network of purine researchers, sharing ideas and data.

In the early years of her work in the Burroughs Wellcome laboratory,

"It was as though the signal was there: 'This is the disease you're going to have to work against.'"

—Gertrude Elion

Elion attended night classes at Brooklyn Polytechnic Institute to complete her Ph.D. It was a long subway ride nightly after work, but she felt she needed this "union card" for scientists working in research. But when the dean called her in and asked her to attend classes full time or leave the program, she told him she could not leave her job—the work was too important to her. For a long time she wasn't sure she had made the right decision.

By 1950, Elion had developed a compound that interfered with the metabolism of leukemia cells in children and young adults with acute leukemia (cancer of the blood). This chemotherapy—the use of drugs to target enemy cells—was not an instant success, however. The drug was tested on animals, and appeared to work beautifully. So two very ill leukemia patients received treatment. One was a woman named J.B., just 23 years old and dying. She recovered, and Elion was ecstatic. But two years later, now married and a mother, J.B. suddenly fell ill again and died. Elion was devastated. With more recent knowledge, J.B.'s physicians would have treated her over a longer period of time, with larger doses, and probably she would still be living today.

Convinced of the ultimate effectiveness of cancer chemotherapy, Elion began working with the biochemistry of the drug she had developed and found she could develop other purine compounds with differing levels of toxicity. She eventually developed and tested more than 100 purine compounds.

During this period, she also discovered she could substitute a sulfur atom for the oxygen atom on a purine molecule. She tested it and found that mice with tumors treated with this drug lived twice as long as those receiving no treatment. Named 6-mercaptopurine, or 6-MP, Elion's drug received the approval of the Federal Drug Administration in 1953. Again, though, remission was temporary, and Elion was torn by the human tragedy of hope dashed eventually by death.

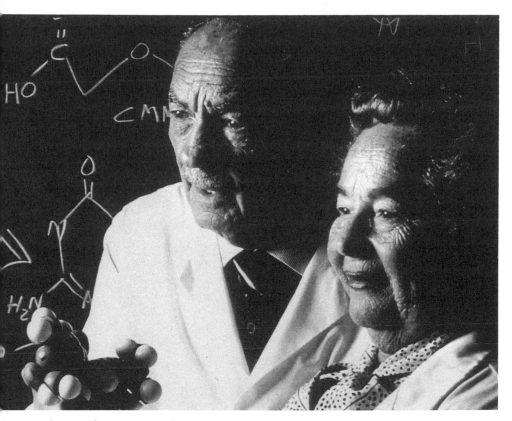

Elion and George Hitchings, Nobel Prize winners, 1988 (Courtesy of Glaxo Wellcome)

"The disappointment with 6-mercaptopurine was that it wasn't good enough," Elion explained. "Until we learned how to use combinations for cancer therapy we weren't curing anybody with single drugs. . . . And for eighteen years of my life, I tried to make 6-mercaptopurine better. I was insistent that this was going to work."

Now used in combination with other drugs, 6-MP has helped change childhood leukemia from a disease of certain death to one where 80 percent of its victims survive.

Even shortly after the approval of 6-MP, despite the early losses, other researchers could see that Elion was on the right track and began testing another way to use 6-MP—to prevent transplant rejection. As we've seen in the work of Burnet and Medawar, physicians had long sought a way to transplant organs from a donor, but the recipient's immune system regularly destroyed the life-giving addition. Today, surgeons can almost routinely remove an ailing kidney, pancreas, liver, heart, lung, or other vital organ, and replace it with one from a donor. But the first successful transplant of a vital whole organ did not occur until 1954, when Joseph E. Murray succeeded in transplanting a kidney from one identical twin to another. It was a landmark achievement, and for this work, Murray won the Nobel Prize in 1990. However, for most people, his accomplishment had one flaw: It depended upon the existence of a donor who was an identical twin, whose body and immune system were so similar to the recipient's that the greatest adversary to success—rejection of the organ by the recipient's body—was virtually overcome.

That's where 6-MP came in. Robert Schwartz of the New England Medical Center found that 6-MP inhibited the growth of antibodies in rabbits. This could mean that, when the body discovers the presence of "non-self," as Frank Macfarlane Burnet put it, 6-MP might be used to suppress the antibodies produced by the immune system. The British transplant surgeon Roy Y. Calne tried using 6-MP as an immuno-suppressant to prevent transplant rejection and found that it worked at first, but then stopped working after a period of time. That's when Gertrude Elion and George H. Hitchings stepped in again, suggesting the use of another purine, azathioprine (Imuran), closely related to 6-MP.

The first use of azathioprine in organ transplant surgery took place at Harvard Medical School in 1960. The recipient was a collie dog named Lollipop, whose kidney transplant succeeded. This success paved the way to the first successful human kidney transplant surgery two years later. Azathioprine continues as a key drug in transplants.

Elion continued to work in this way, using one discovery to open the doors to others. Every time she discovered something new about the way a compound worked or the way a nucleic acid was synthesized, she used that knowledge to explore all the implications. "This kind of leverage technique, where every time you get a piece of information you use it as a tool to pull more information out—that was one of the key elements of her strategy," her colleague James Burchall told one interviewer. She used this technique—starting with George Hitchings's methods and pushing ever forward—to develop an amazing number of compounds. Each drug attacked a different part of the nucleic acid's metabolism.

In 1966 Elion synthesized allopurinol. Actually a spin-off from her effort to make the effect of 6-MP last longer, she discovered that an enzyme she had hoped to use to retard the breakdown of 6-MP instead reduced the body's production of uric acid. Excessive production of uric acid can cause crystal deposits in the joints, which produce the painful swelling of the feet and hands in gout. Deposits can also take the form of kidney stones and cause blockage and damage to the kidneys and urinary system. Large amounts of uric acid are often produced by cancer chemotherapy and radiation therapy, causing similar problems for patients under these treatments. Allopurinol could help this problem—inhibiting the enzyme xanthine oxidase and blocking the formation of uric acid in the last step of the metabolic pathway. Elion was delighted. Before allopurinol, more than 10,000 people suffering from gout died from kidney blockage each year in the United States. Now there was a viable remedy. In 1963 the first test was made on a gout sufferer, a night watchman. His symptoms disappeared and he returned to work within three days.

Ten years later, researchers discovered that allopurinol was an effective treatment for Leshmaniasis disease, which is rampant in South America. Elion campaigned to get Burroughs Wellcome to make the drug available there. As Thomas Krenitsky, research vice president at Burroughs Wellcome, asserted in the 1990s, "In fifty years, Trudy Elion will have done more cumulatively for the human condition than Mother Teresa."

Elion became head of the Department of Experimental Therapy at Burroughs Wellcome in 1967, when Hitchings retired from active research to become vice president of research. Now she was on her own. During this period, Elion went back to the drug she had developed in 1948, the forerunner of 6-MP. Called 2,6-diaminopurine, it had proved too toxic to be useful. But in 1968 she heard the news that certain nucleotide compounds, arabinosides, had been shown to inhibit the growth of viruses. The trouble was that arabinosides didn't last long before they broke down. "The information started a train of thought," Elion later recalled. Maybe artificial arabinosides would last longer, and would still fight the viruses. Finally, after many complications, in 1974 she announced the synthesis of a new compound, acyclovir. It was the first drug ever to work against viruses, and it is still used to fight herpes viruses, including the varicella zoster virus, which causes chickenpox and shingles. The drug has proved particularly useful in helping people with inadequate immune systems, such as those with leukemia, cancer, transplanted organs, or AIDS (acquired immune deficiency syndrome).

"In fifty years, Trudy Elion will have done more cumulatively for the human condition than Mother Teresa."

—Thomas Krenitsky

Acyclovir, according to Elion, was her "final jewel. . . . It was a real breakthrough in antiviral research.

That such a thing was possible wasn't even imagined up until then."

In 1970, Burroughs Wellcome moved from suburban New York to Research Triangle Park in North Carolina. It was a big change for a native New Yorker. Elion had never married, although she had planned to at one time, in the late 1930s. Leonard had been a statistics major at City College, obtained a fellowship to study abroad, and had returned. But he became gravely ill with acute bacterial endocarditis—a strep-tococcus infection of the heart valves and lining—and died suddenly. No one else could ever measure up in Elion's eyes, and she never gave marriage another thought. But her home had always been New York, and she loved the Metropolitan Opera, to which she always had season tickets. She moved all her memorabilia into a two-story condominium in North Carolina, but, since she always loved to travel, she kept her opera subscription.

Despite her intense work schedule, Elion always contin-ued to hold close the family ties that were so important in her childhood and early years. She remained close to her brother Herbert, and became a doting aunt to his children and grandchildren, making frequent trips to California, where he established a bioengineering and communications engineering company. When she traveled to Stockholm for the Nobel award ceremony, she took with her 11 members of her family.

Elion retired from Burroughs Wellcome in 1983, but continued to consult in the lab there, also teaching research methods to medical students at nearby Duke University. "In a sense," she once remarked, "my career appears to have come full circle from my early days of being a teacher to now sharing my experience in research with the new generations of scientists." She has also served on the national committee for reviewing procedures for the approval of new cancer and AIDS drugs; on the National Cancer Advisory Board; and on World Health Organization committees on three tropical diseases: filariasis, river blindness, and malaria. Elion has also served on boards of the National Cancer Institute, the American Cancer Society, and the Multiple Sclerosis Society.

In all, Elion holds 45 patents based on her 39 years at Burroughs Wellcome. Following her retirement, colleagues at Burroughs Wellcome (now Glaxo Wellcome) used the methods that she and Hitchings perfected to develop azidothymidine (AZT), the first drug approved by the U.S. Food and Drug Administration for treating AIDS patients. The legacy continues.

By 1988, when she and Hitchings became Nobel laureates, Elion had become an internationally recognized leader in the field of purine antimetabolites for the treatment of cancer—which she likes to call the "purine path to chemotherapy."

As the Nobel committee explained, the contribution made by Elion and Hitchings goes beyond the value of the specific drugs they developed. They have created a new

> rational approach to the discovery of new drugs, based upon basic scientific studies of biochemical and physiological processes. As a result, a new era in drug research was born which offers promise for the development of new therapeutic strategies for the treatment of illnesses against which existing drugs are either unsatisfactory or simply do not exist.

Elion has long since made up for dropping out of the Brooklyn Polytechnic Institute Ph.D. program, having received numerous honorary doctorates. And, in addition to the Nobel Prize and induction into the National Inventors' Hall of Fame, she has received numerous other awards in her field and was elected to the National Academy of Sciences and the National Women's Hall of Fame. But for Elion, these are not her most important achievements. "The Nobel Prize is fine," she told *The New York Times Magazine*, "but the drugs I've developed are rewards in themselves."

In her office, Elion has a drawerful of letters that she keeps to remind herself of these rewards—a drawerful of heartfelt thank yous from people whose loved ones' lives were saved or whose own lives were saved. These letters are from real people, telling their life stories, filled with phrases like, "Your hard work and relentless dedication were involved in the cure of my son's reticulum cell sarcoma when he was fifteen years old." Or, in the words of a father whose son was saved by 6-MP: ". . . it is with inexpressible gratitude for having contributed to the saving of one human life so very dear to me and so many other human lives that I write to say to you in the simplest, and hence, the most profound and sincere of terms, thank you!"

Chronology

January 23, 1918	Gertrude Belle Elion is born in New York City
1937	Graduates from Hunter College *summa cum laude*
1941	Receives master of science degree, New York University
1941–42	Teaches high school chemistry and physics
1944	Joins Wellcome Research Laboratories (now Glaxo Wellcome)
1951	Elion discovers 6-MP, the first effective compound against childhood leukemia, approved by FDA in 1953

1962	First successful human kidney transplant, using azathioprine (Imuran), developed by Elion
1966	Invention of allopurinol (Zyloprim) for the treatment of gout
1967	Becomes head of experimental therapy at Burroughs Wellcome
1983	Elion retires from Burroughs Wellcome
1984	Using Elion's and Hitchings's methods, Elion's laboratory at Burroughs Wellcome develops azidothymidine (AZT), the first drug approved to treat AIDS
1988	Nobel Prize for physiology or medicine, shared with George H. Hitchings
1991	Awarded National Medal of Science; inducted into the National Inventors Hall of Fame

Further Reading

Bailey, Martha J. *American Women in Science: A Biographical Dictionary*. Santa Barbara: ABC-CLIO, Inc., 1994.

Bouton, Katherine. "The Nobel Pair." *The New York Times Magazine*, January 29, 1989.

Colburn, Don. "The Pathway to the Prize." *The Washington Post*, October 25, 1988.

Elion, Gertrude. "The Purine Path to Chemotherapy." *Science*, April 7, 1989.

Hitchings, George H., and Gertrude B. Elion. "Layer on Layer." *Cancer Research* 45, June 1985, pp. 2415–20.

Holloway, Marguerite. "The Satisfaction of Delayed Gratification." *Scientific American*, October 1991, pp. 40–44.

Marshall, Liz. "Gertrude Belle Elion, 1918– ," in *Notable Twentieth-Century Scientists*, edited by Emily J. McMurray, Vol. I, pp. 582–585. New York: Gale Research, Inc., 1995.

McGrayne, Sharon Bertsch. *Nobel Prize Women in Science: Their Lives, Struggles, and Momentous Discoveries*. New York: Carol Publishing Group, 1992.

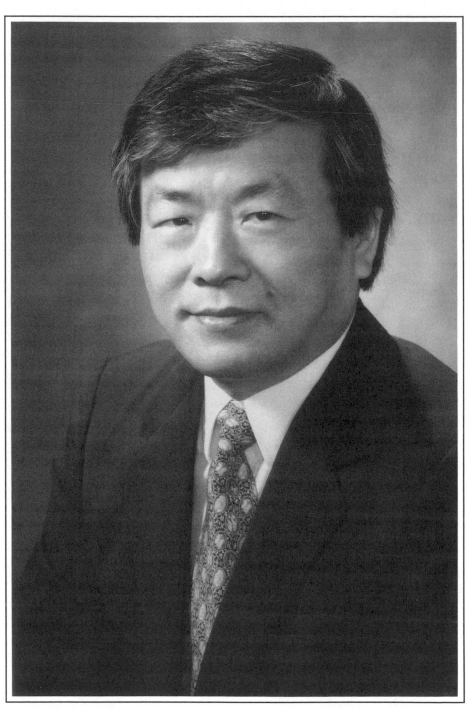

Susumu Tonegawa (Courtesy of the Massachusetts Institute of Technology)

Susumu Tonegawa

"TOO MANY CHAINS—
TOO FEW GENES,"
THE MYSTERY OF ANTIBODY
DIVERSITY (1939–   )

As the final months of 1970 approached, 31-year-old Susumu Tonegawa [toh nay GAH wah] reached a perplexing crossroads. Newly graduated from the University of Kyoto, he had come to San Diego, California, in 1963—but not to soak up the sun on the sandy California beaches, or visit the attractions of nearby Mexico. Instead, he had spent the past seven years learning everything he could about molecular biology, first in San Diego and then in La Jolla, California.

His work in molecular biology had gone well. He had completed his Ph.D. and postdoctoral studies. And he had co-authored several published scientific papers. But his United States visa was about to expire at the end of December, and he would have to leave the United States for at least two years. The question that continually haunted him now was, Where to next?

That's when a timely letter arrived from Renato Dulbecco. Dulbecco, with whom Tonegawa had worked at the Salk Institute in La Jolla, had been doing important work on monoclonal (derived from one cell) antibodies (which would earn Dulbecco a Nobel Prize five years later). The older man was traveling in Europe, and he had what he seemed to think was exciting news for Tonegawa. The Institute of Immunology in Basel, Switzerland, he wrote, needed a molecular biologist.

But Tonegawa wasn't sure. Without any background in immunology, how would he, with a freshly minted doctorate in molecular biology, have a chance at a position at the newly formed Swiss institute? But time was short, so he set aside his misgivings and applied anyway. And he was accepted. So by January 1971, Susumu Tonegawa had set out for the little town on the Rhine—no closer to his home in Japan—to begin the work that would lead him, within 16 years, to become the first Japanese recipient of the Nobel Prize in physiology or medicine.

Susumu Tonegawa was born September 5, 1939, in Nagoya, a large city about 150 miles southwest of Tokyo, Japan. He was the second of four children born to Tsutomu Tonegawa and Miyoko Masuko (his mother's name prior to her marriage). His father worked for a textile company as an engineer, and the work required frequent moves among rural towns in different parts of the country. The Tonegawa children enjoyed the open space and freedom of country life, but eventually, the two oldest children—Susumu and his older brother—were sent to live with an uncle in Tokyo. There the two boys could attend the prestigious Hibiya High School, and during these years young Tonegawa became keenly interested in chemistry. He decided he would pursue his studies at Kyoto University. But the tough entrance examination proved a stumbling block the first time he took it. Finally, in 1959, at the age of 20, he succeeded in gaining entrance to the university, where he majored in chemistry.

At this particular time, in the 50s and early 60s, the field of molecular biology was just emerging. The new research area especially attracted scientists with backgrounds in both chemistry and biology, since molecular biology required an understanding of how molecules react (the realm of the chemist) and of how living things function (the realm of biology). In 1953, Francis Crick and James Watson discovered the structure of one of the most fundamental biological molecules, DNA or deoxyribonucleic acid. Essentially, Crick and Watson's exciting discovery revealed the mechanism by which genetic information is stored in molecules. The sequence of molecules along the strand of atoms in the DNA molecule, they discovered, forms a code. And this DNA code transmits information about the cellular form and function to a biological cell's offspring.

Crick and Watson's discovery was one of the most important of the 20th century, and it transformed the field of biology. Exciting possibilities opened up for looking at biological processes from fresh perspectives, and as an undergraduate Tonegawa developed a keen interest in molecular biology. He earned his bachelor's degree in chemistry at Kyoto in 1963 and began his graduate studies there, working for two months under Itaru Watanabe at the University of Kyoto's Institute for Virus Research. But Watanabe saw that Tonegawa held promise and recognized the limitations of the Institute's facilities for molecular biology. He suggested to Tonegawa that he make a move to a school with more extensive equipment for studies in molecular biology.

Just a few months later, in the fall of 1963, Tonegawa crossed the Pacific to begin graduate studies in molecular biology at the University of California at San Diego. There he studied in the Biology Department under Masaki Hayashi, with whom he published three scientific papers between 1966 and 1970 on genetic transcription and molecular biology. (Genetic transcription is the process by which genetic information is transferred from a DNA molecule to messenger RNA, the form of RNA or ribonucleic acid that serves as a template, or pattern, for protein synthesis.) In 1968 he received his Ph.D. in biology, and he stayed on to pursue seven months of postdoctoral work with Hayashi from September 1968 to April 1969. In May 1969 he moved over to the Salk Institute for Biological Studies at nearby La Jolla, where he worked under Renato Dulbecco from May 1969 to December 1970. There he conducted postdoctoral studies on genetic transcription in simian virus 40 (SV40).

At the end of this period of intensive study, Tonegawa received his appointment as molecular biologist at the newly established Institute of Immunology in Basel, where he arrived in January 1971. In Basel, as he would later declare in his Nobel Prize lecture, he found himself "surrounded by immunologists." It turned out to be an invigorating environment, for here he began the work that eventually led him to the Nobel Prize.

The body's immune system is an integrated group of organs, tissues, cells, and cell products—such as antibodies—that help the body distinguish between what is "self" and "nonself," as Macfarlane Burnet put it. It's the body's method of protecting itself against foreign and potentially harmful substances or organisms, which have come to be called antigens. Immunologists study the immune system and how it works, examining the behavior of invading antigens and the ways an organism fights off these invaders. In vertebrates, including humans, an individual can develop a specific antibody to defend against a specific invading antigen—including toxins, bacteria, foreign blood cells, and the cells of transplanted organs. This was the principle that Salk and Sabin used when they developed their polio vaccines.

Now Tonegawa brought his skills as a microbiologist to immunology. He wanted to take a look at what was happening between antibodies and antigens at the molecular level.

"I felt from the beginning that I could contribute to resolving this question by applying the recently invented techniques of molecular biology," Tonegawa later wrote.

Some groundwork had already been laid. In the 1950s and 1960s, Rodney R. Porter and Gerald M. Edelman had outlined the general structure of an antibody molecule. They had showed that antibodies are Y-shaped protein molecules that consist of two amino-acid chains combined. When foreign substances—including bacterial and viral infections—invade the body, the antibodies disable them by attaching themselves to the antigens by the tips of the branches of the Y. But the fit must be exact.

Rescarchers also knew that antibodies originate in a particular class of white blood cells, called B lymphocytes, or B cells. As Tonegawa later wrote,

> Their basic mode of action can be understood in terms of the clonal selection theory proposed 30 years ago by Sir Macfarlane Burnet. As each B cell matures in the bone marrow, it becomes committed to the synthesis of antibodies that recognize a specific antigen, or molecular pattern.

Biologists had also known for a long time that a vertebrate can produce millions, even billions, of antibodies, without the presence of an antigen of any kind—a very useful adaptation, since the potential number of types of antigens is enormous.

Each B cell retains the antibodies it has created. They are displayed on the surface as receptor molecules, bound to the membrane of the B cell. Each antibody is designed to recognize a specific antigenic marker—a comparatively small pattern of molecular structure. Then, once an antigen comes along and becomes attached to the tips of the Y-shaped antibody, the B cell becomes stimulated to multiply. This is the clonal-selection process Burnet was talking about, with many clones produced as the result of a single infection.

The problem was that the number of genes available to generate the antibody's amino-acid chains was far fewer than the number of chains produced. So the question was: How? How did the body manage to adapt by producing this enormous number of antibodies?

The prevailing theory at the time, known as the "germ line" theory, maintained that all the genes necessary to make every antigen were part of the genetic code. But the problem with this theory was that, if true, then the genetic coding for all the body's antibodies had to be pre-stored. Yet the total number of genes in the human genetic system—which is among the most complex—is 100,000. How could so many come from so few? Additionally, as Tonegawa later put it,

"The genetic side of antibody research was a complete mystery to us all when Tonegawa started his work. He was the only player in the field between 1976 and 1978."

—Karolinska Institute President Bengt Samuelsson, 1987

"The accepted dogma had been that genes (regulating the immune system) do not move around."

As Tonegawa wrote in his article on "The Molecules of the Immune System," in *Scientific American*, "The critical event in mounting an immune response is the recognition of chemical markers that distinguish self from nonself. The molecules entrusted with this task are proteins whose most intriguing property is their variability of structure." This became the key subject of his exploration.

Recognition of the chemical markers, Tonegawa saw, is performed by proteins that have an enormously variable structure. As he later wrote, generally all molecules of a given protein made by an individual are "absolutely identical: they have the same sequence of amino acids." At most, there might be two versions—one version specified by the set of genes inherited from the mother; the other dictated by the father's genes. But that's all. "The recognition proteins of the immune system, in contrast, come in millions or perhaps billions of slightly different forms." Because there are so many different forms, the recognition proteins are able to recognize and target a huge number of specific target patterns.

Tonegawa was able to pinpoint the genetic mechanisms responsible for this diversity. He worked with mouse cells and was able to show that, during the development of the B-lymphocyte cell, the genes coding for antibodies get shuffled at random. As a result, the mature cell contains a cluster of functional genes that are specific to that cell.

But that's only part of the diversification available to antibodies. Unlike other cells, the immune system cells have "hot spots," particularly sensitive gene fragments which arrange themselves with other fragments to produce millions of different antibodies. Each antibody molecule is composed of four protein chains, all of which are highly variable in the terminal portion of the Y. Multiply this potential for diversity by the huge number of lymphocytes in the body, "each with its own combination of functional antibody-producing genes," and you begin to get a very large number of possibilities.

According to this evidence DNA is not an inactive archive of information. It can be—and routinely is—altered during an individual's life span. This cutting and joining of gene sequences during the synthesis of antibodies, Tonegawa pointed out, is not just an incidental feature of the genetic process. It is essential to the way the immune system operates.

From these insights Tonegawa and his colleagues, including Niels Jerne and Nobumichi Hozumi, developed the "somatic theory" of the immune system, showing how only a few hundred gene fragments, which individually code for only parts of antibody proteins, can combine in millions, even billions, of ways to produce the enormous flexibility of the immune response. As a result, these proteins, the recognizers of foreign invaders, according to Tonegawa, are the most diverse proteins known.

With Hozumi, Tonegawa also discovered that the DNA segments that undergo rearrangement are separated by seemingly inactive (noncoding) strands of DNA, now known as introns. (An intron is a section of a gene that does not function in coding for protein synthesis.)

Jean L. Marx, writing in *Science*, observed that Tonegawa's work has far-reaching significance: "One unexpected consequence of the antibody gene research was new information about the possible causes of cancer especially the blood cancers known as lymphomas and leukemias." Tonegawa's work demonstrating the dynamic character of genetic rearrangement in the immune system is considered a key to future insights concerning the causes of some cancers. Some researchers postulate that introns may conceivably break off in the normal process of genetic transcription—when messenger RNA heads out to the ribosome to direct the production of protein. Introns are known to cut themselves out during this process. Do they sometimes float off to cause problems elsewhere in the system? This is a distinct possibility.

Tonegawa continued his work at Basel for 10 years, until 1981, when he received an invitation from Salvador Luria at MIT to return to the United States as professor of biology in the Center for Cancer Research and Department of Biology there. He accepted. There, he continued the work he began in Switzerland, and has played a key role in explaining how the receptors on T cells function. T cells are another important

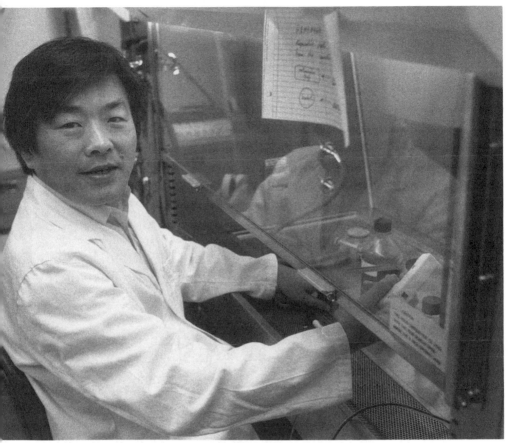

Tonegawa in his laboratory (Courtesy of the Massachusetts Institute of Technology)

component of the immune system, vital to the fight against viruses.

In 1992, Tonegawa and his colleagues at MIT identified, for the first time, a specific gene in mice that has an effect on the ability to learn. Such a specific link in mammals between a particular gene and a learning deficit shed new light on the molecular mechanisms of learning and memory. The *New York Times* called this research "the first step toward discovering the entire repertoire of genes that affect brain function."

The group focused specifically on spatial learning—the ability of an organism to find precise locations in a complex environment. Using a relatively new genetic engineering technique, they eliminated a specific gene from mice—the gene that encodes a molecular component of the hippocampus, a part of the brain thought to be necessary for learning the relative location of objects in space. When the researchers placed these mice in a common behavioral test maze, they were unable to learn the location of objects placed in the maze. Normal mice had no problem with the exercise.

Tonegawa and his colleagues said that the test mice had difficulty because the cells of the hippocampus lacked long-term potentiation (LTP), the ability to stabilize cell-to-cell transfer of information. Their data seemed to substantiate a hypothesis held for some time by scientists that learning initiates changes in the strength of the connections among the brain cells that process the information to be remembered.

The research raises hopes, as Charles Stevens of the Salk Institute pointed out, that the knowledge gained in the ongoing research may lead to changes in clinical applications that will help stroke and trauma victims recover. It also provides insights expected to be valuable in the treatment of epilepsy and chronic anxiety.

In 1994, MIT announced the establishment of a new Center for Learning and Memory (CLM) to explore the biology of learning and memory, naming Susumu Tonegawa as its director. Interdisciplinary in nature, the CLM represents a coordinated effort of the MIT departments of biology and of brain and cognitive sciences, as well as computer scientists, mathematicians, chemists, and physicists. At the time of his appointment,

"In some respects neurobiology stands now at a point where biology as a whole stood four decades ago."

—Susumu Tonegawa, 1994

Tonegawa commented, "In some respects neurobiology stands now at a point where biology as a whole stood four decades ago. Many scientists believe that neuroscience, the study of how our brain functions, is the most exciting branch of science in the rest of this century and beyond." He envisioned not only many health benefits from understanding of functions such as learning and memory, but there is also, he said, "an exciting sense that the crossing of what has been called science's last frontier—explaining the nature of the human mind—is for the first time a realistic prospect."

On September 28, 1985 Susumu Tonegawa married Mayumi Yoshinari, then a student at MIT studying the brain and cognitive science. The Tonegawas have three children. The author of some 162 papers, Tonegawa works long hours, often far into the night, and colleagues describe him as "an aggressive, driven, and brilliant researcher." Although he makes his home in Massachusetts, he has always retained his Japanese citizenship, and in 1984 he received the award of the Bunkakunsho Order of Culture from the Emperor of Japan.

Tonegawa has received numerous honors and awards worldwide for his work, from immunology societies, governments, and professional organizations in Japan, Switzerland, Germany, Brazil, Israel, the United States, and Canada. In 1986, Tonegawa was elected to the U.S. National Academy of Sciences, considered one of the highest honors that can be accorded a scientist in the United States. Also in 1986, he received the Bristol Myers Award for Distinguished Achievement in Cancer Research. In 1988, he was made Howard Hughes Medical Institute Investigator at MIT.

When he received the Nobel Prize in 1987—one of only four nonshared Nobel Prizes for physiology or medicine awarded since 1960—Tonegawa expressed surprise. Sources in Sweden, however, indicated that he had long been a front runner. Speaking for Sweden's Karolinska Institute, its president, Bengt Samuelsson, said, "The genetic side of antibody research was a complete mystery to us all when Tonegawa started his work. He was the only player in the field between 1976 and 1978. The work was truly unique." Tonegawa's research, he said, provided doctors with an important basic tool for research into finding cures for many diseases.

Chronology

September 5, 1939	Susumu Tonegawa is born in Nagoya, Japan
1963	Graduates from the University of Kyoto; begins graduate studies at University of California at San Diego
1968	Receives Ph.D. in biology
1968–70	Post-doctoral work at UC San Diego and the Salk Institute in La Jolla, California
1971	Begins work as a molecular biologist at the Institute of Immunology in Basel, Switzerland
1981	Becomes professor of biology in the Center for Cancer Research and Department of Biology at Massachusetts Institute of Technology
1985	Marries Mayumi Yoshinari
1987	Nobel Prize in physiology or medicine
1988	Awarded position of investigator at the Howard Hughes Medical Institute
1992	Announces discovery of a gene linked to learning deficiency in mice
1994	Named director of the MIT Center for Learning and Memory

Further Reading

Daintith, John, et al., eds. *Biographical Encyclopedia of Scientists, 2nd Edition*. Bristol: Institute of Physics Publishing, 1994.

McGuire, Paula, editor. *Nobel Prize Winners Supplement, 1987–1991*. New York: H.W. Wilson Co., 1992, pp. 136–139.

Newton, David E. "Susumu Tonegawa, 1939– : Japanese molecular biologist," *Notable Twentieth-Century Scientists*. Emily J. McMurray, Editor. New York: Gale Research, Inc., 1995, Vol. 4, pp. 2040–2042.

Tonegawa, Susumu. "The Molecules of the Immune System." *Scientific American*, October 1985, p. 122, ff.

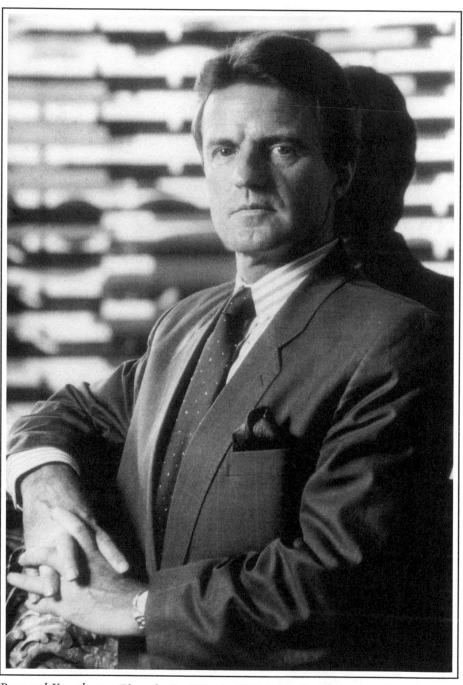

Bernard Kouchner (Photo by José Nicolas/SIPA Press, Courtesy of the Consulate of France)

Bernard Kouchner

FIGHTING DISASTER WITH MEDICAL RELIEF (1939–)

O n the outskirts of Khost, Afghanistan, in December 1987, 18 doctors and nurses had gathered together a herd of sure-footed, sinewy ponies. Their purpose: to ferry the pieces of their field hospital and its staff over the mountain pass to the aid of the wounded. These are the "troops" of Doctors Without Borders, among them Bernard Kouchner [koosh nehr], the doctor who founded this guerrilla-style group of medical revolutionaries. On this occasion they have traveled 800 kilometers through the war-torn mountains of Afghanistan. They have often had to move at night, slipping through empty, eerie villages, gliding like ghosts past threatening gun installations.

Now, dressed in the clothing of local peasants, they are approaching Khost, currently under siege by the mujahideen, defended by the Russians. But their peasant clothing no longer works as a good disguise. They are trapped. Russian guns are poised within easy range, and the shells are hitting much too close. They must make a run for it, across open ground. They take off in a tumbling chaos of galloping, hooves flying, horses stumbling. Finally they reach the other side, where the

> mujahideen in their red beards are waiting. Miracu-
> lously, no one is hurt, and the supplies they have brought
> are intact. The doctors have crossed the borders again.

Bernard Kouchner has many sides. He's a well-educated intellectual, a charming socialite, a dandy, and a wealthy and powerful figure in European politics. He is also a committed physician—a man obsessed with a vision for a better world, a world where children can grow up healthy and where people of all nations have a chance for a life free of poverty, pain, disease, and war. In his battle for this vision, Bernard Kouchner has fought literally on the front lines of the world's wars, rolling up his sleeves and hoisting medical supplies on his shoulders, bandaging the wounded, and ducking flying bullets with the toughest and bravest. He has also become a powerful, charismatic, and effective force for compassionate international public action.

Born November 1, 1939 in Avignon, France, Kouchner is a medical doctor who has taken on the world as his practice. As he was growing up in the suburbs of Paris, Kouchner found intellectual stimulation in the writings of the French existentialist philosopher Jean-Paul Sartre and the poet-novelist Louis Aragon, among others. As a young man he was an activist, he says, who liked sports cars. In 1964 he finished his medical degree, becoming certified as a gastroenterologist.

Greatly influenced by Sartre and other existentialists, Kouchner was drawn to issues of social injustice. Basic to existential philosophy are the ideas that human beings exist in a universe that is indifferent and alien, and that consequently individuals must choose the acts and direction of their lives and assume responsibility for those choices. These ideas had an enormous impact on Kouchner. Although an activist, he was critical of what he saw as empty "activist" gestures, such as the student and worker revolts of May 1968 in France, which he called an "exercise in style." For him the deepest issue of the late 1960s and 1970s was the tragedy taking place in eastern Nigeria, where Biafra had seceded from the larger federation in 1967. Nigeria refused to recognize the independent state of Biafra and began to wage the bloodiest civil war ever fought on the continent of Africa up to that time. That's when Kouchner joined the International Committee for the Red Cross, which was recruiting volunteers. Kouchner and several of his friends left France for Biafra in the summer of 1968. But idealistic hopes of bringing help were quickly disappointed. The hospitals were crowded with three or four times more patients than beds, and the wounded arrived from the front lines by the truckload. As he watched helplessly, Kouchner began to feel strongly that the Nigerian government was attempting to eradicate an entire people. Nigerian troops even bombed and attacked the hospital where Kouchner and his colleagues were trying to mend the sick and wounded.

Finally, he spoke out to his fellow physicians. "We are facing a mass murder," he said. He was trying to save victims of the intense civil war taking place there, but he felt hampered by the Red Cross charter, which prevents intervention by volunteers in national policy. Kouchner found himself unable to stand by neutrally in the face of civil conflicts resulting in horrifying bloodshed and desperate human agony such as he witnessed in Nigeria. In the end, he left the Red Cross and called for a press conference on his return to

"If a child is being beaten in the apartment next to yours, you can call the cops, but you also have a right to break down the door."

—Bernard Kouchner

Paris in 1969 to discuss the events he had witnessed. It was then he began to think about a different way of doing things.

In 1970 he and his colleague Max Recamier banded with about 50 others to begin organizing courses in emergency medicine and relief missions. Later that year he joined others in his group to travel to Peru to help victims of an earthquake and also cooperated with the Red Cross in Jordan after the Black September massacre of Palestinians.

In 1971 Kouchner founded an independent organization, Médecins sans Frontières (Doctors Without Borders), a group of doctors who ignore national boundaries and don't restrict themselves to healing the wounded. Not bound by a credo of neutrality, when these doctors saw civil rights abuses, they spoke out. They functioned on a shoestring budget with financial support from a pharmaceutical publication, but were able to send teams to Nicaragua in 1972 where an earthquake had left many people homeless and wounded, and 6,000 dead. In 1975, MSF teams went to Lebanon to aid victims of a vicious civil war, in April of that year to Vietnam following the fall of Saigon, and in 1976 to Turkey following a devastating earthquake.

However, Kouchner liked doing things with a flourish and courted the attention of the media. Because some of his colleagues disapproved, or were envious, of his charismatic approach, Kouchner left the MSF in 1980 to found a similar group, Médecins du Monde (Doctors of the World). Between them, the two groups have continued to travel the world, bringing much-needed food, medical supplies, and hope to those in distress. They can be found in the Middle East, Africa, Southeast Asia, and Latin America.

Kouchner's basic credo is that he or any representative of any nation has the right to intervene. The key concept is to relieve suffering for those stricken by disasters (whether natural or man-made) and plagued by poverty. "If a child is being beaten in the apartment next to yours, you can call the cops," Kouchner explains, "but you also have a right to break down the door." Kouchner's point of view violates some key principles of international diplomacy, which respect national sovereignty and operate on the premise that I'll stay off your back, if you'll stay off mine. His ideas are radical, and not everyone agrees with them, but no one can question that he gets results.

More recently, Kouchner has wielded his influence at higher levels. From 1988 to 1993, he served in several high-level capacities in the national government of France—culminating in two years as Minister of Health and Humanitarian Affairs. From this platform, he became France's ambassador for health, peace, and cooperation, making countless high-profile visits on humanitarian missions to aid victims of natural, economic, and political disasters. The early winter of 1989 saw him escorting wounded Muslims to safety in war-torn Beirut. In January 1990 he flew again to Beirut after clashes erupted between warring Christian factions. In July 1990 he aided Albanian refugees, and in the spring of 1991, France sent Kouchner to Iraq to arrange aid for Kurdish refugees. In 1992, when ethnic violence in Sarajevo was reaching outrageous proportions, the French once again sent Kouchner to open up an air bridge into the city despite the Serbian artillery still posted in the hills. In February 1993, he secured an agreement among Bosnia's warring parties for a prisoner swap involving 216 inmates.

In 1994 Kouchner was elected to the European Parliament and since divides his time between Brussels,

"... the international community has a right to make humanitarian interventions that ignore national sovereignty when grave violations of human rights exist."

—William Pfaff,
Los Angeles Times columnist

where the Parliament meets, and his home in Paris, where he lives with TV journalist Christine Ockrent, with whom he has a son, Alexandre. He also has three other children—Julien, Camille, and Antoine—from his former marriage to university educator Evelyne Pisier.

Despite an early reputation for heading a group, as he once put it, of "dangerous madmen," Kouchner has received many accolades. For his humanitarian work he received the prestigious Dag Hammarskjöld prize in 1979, the Athinai Prize of the Alexander Onassis Foundation in 1981, and the Europa Prize in 1984. He is a figure of considerable stature, with a degree of leverage rarely enjoyed by physicians on the international political scene, and his global view of human rights has begun to gain supporters. As *Los Angeles Times* syndicated columnist William Pfaff put it in July 1992:

> Nothing would have happened without France's initiatives, which reflected the developing conviction of France, promoted by the minister of health, Bernard Kouchner, among others, that the international community has a right to make humanitarian interventions that ignore national sovereignty when grave violations of human rights exist.

For Kouchner, the risks and drawbacks never outweigh the need to save suffering victims of the world instead of sitting by and looking for reasons to do nothing. As he likes to say, "You invent the rights of tomorrow."

Chronology

November 1, 1939	Bernard Kouchner is born in Avignon, France
1964	Receives medical degree

1971	Founds Doctors Without Borders (Médecins sans Frontières)
1979	Receives Hammarskjöld prize
1980	Founds Doctors of the World (Médecins du Monde) and serves as president until 1984
1988–1993	Serves in several high-level capacities in the national government of France—culminating in two years as Minister of Health and Humanitarian Action; organizes humanitarian missions to aid victims of natural, economic, and political disasters
1993	Creates the Foundation for Humanitarian Action
1994	Elected to the European Parliament

Further Reading

1993 Current Biography Yearbook, pp. 323–327.
The New York Times Magazine, pp. 30 ff., July 28, 1991.
Dickey, Christopher. "France's Guerrilla Doctor." *Vanity Fair* 56: pp. 92 ff., April 1993.
"Students Without Borders." *Harvard Public Health Review*, Spring 1995.
Who's Who in France, 1992–93.

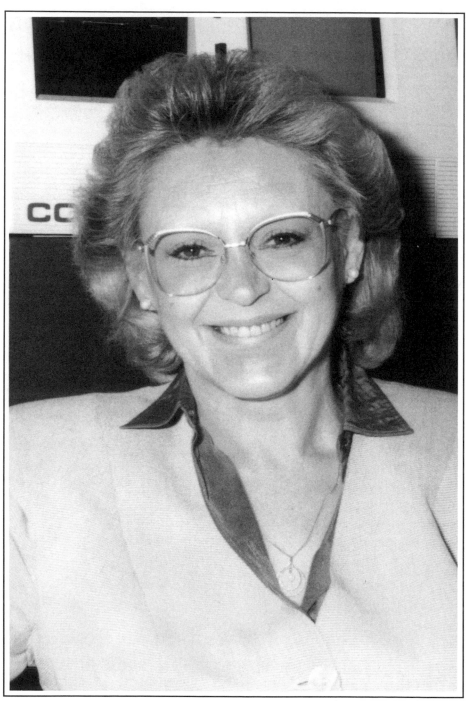

Françoise Barré-Sinoussi (Courtesy of the Institut Pasteur)

Françoise Barré-Sinoussi

THE VIRUS THAT CAUSES AIDS
(1947–   )

AIDS has become the most challenging health issue of the last quarter century. Acquired Immuno Deficiency Syndrome was not even heard of in 1975, and yet by 1995, AIDS rivaled all previous epidemics in degree of challenge and complexity. Reports began filtering in during the late 70s, but the first real evidence anyone noticed came in 1981. A technologist at the Centers for Disease Control in Atlanta noticed that an unusual number of requests had come in for a drug used to treat a very rare skin cancer, Kaposi's sarcoma. Most of the patients were young, white males, most of them homosexual. Previously, Kaposi's sarcoma had been found mostly in Africa and among older Jewish and Italian men in Europe and the United States. At the same time a second rare disease kept turning up among young homosexuals, a pneumonia caused by *Pneumocystis carinii*. A cancer called non-Hodgkin's lymphoma was a third. What all these patients had in common was a severe depletion of T cells, a type of white blood cell that's a key part of the immune system. By the end of the year, the CDC had recorded over 300 cases in the United States of what began to emerge as a new disease—of which these rare diseases turned out to be only symptoms.

By 1985, in the United States 6,681 people had died from AIDS and 8,210 new cases had turned up. By 1991, the statistics had surged to 30,579 deaths and 43,701 new cases—some 65,000 new cases by 1994. In the seven-year span between 1985 and 1991, a total of 166,211 people died of AIDS.

Once infected, an individual can carry the AIDS virus for years before even becoming ill from the disease. During those years many transmissions can take place, spreading the virus to others. An epidemic of Ebola fever in 1995, by contrast, burned itself out in Zaire within a matter of months. There had been no outbreak of the fever, which is caused by the Ebola virus, for 19 years, when suddenly people in the densely populated town of Kikwit began dying within days of becoming ill. The symptoms—which include diarrhea and massive bleeding from all body openings—could allow the virus to spread easily from patient to patient, and no drug had any effect. Of 315 people infected within a six-month period, 244 died, but this swift, high mortality rate defeated the virus in the end. The Ebola epidemic had burned itself out partly because it destroyed its hosts so quickly. Once quarantined, they often had little opportunity to pass the virus on to other hosts. AIDS, however, has not burned itself out.

But AIDS is also very complicated biologically—caused by a virus that comes in many different, and constantly varying, forms. Thousands of workers—from laboratory scientists to public health officials to evolutionary biologists—are striving to find ways to combat the inroads of this pernicious disease. Among them, one of the most prominent—and yet one of the least well-known—is Françoise Barré-Sinoussi of the

> Pasteur Institute in Paris. Vivacious and energetic, Barré-Sinoussi has produced a body of laboratory work in the field of retrovirus microbiology that can only be described as mind-boggling.

Françoise Claire Sinoussi, the daughter of Roger Sinoussi, a building inspector, and Jeanine Fau Sinoussi, was born in Paris, in the 19th district (*19e arrondissement*), one hot summer day, July 30, 1947—two years after the end of World War II. This northeastern district on the outskirts of Paris, bisected by the Canal de l'Ourcq and often described as unfashionable, was for many years the home of slaughter-houses and cattle yards; and the German tanks and bombers had not been kind to this region of Paris during the war. But postwar Paris was an exciting city to grow up in, and appropriately enough, the district where Françoise Sinoussi was born now boasts a science museum in the vast Parc de Villettes on the edge of the city.

Françoise completed her secondary education at the Lycée Bergson and attended the prestigious University of Paris, where she received her diploma in 1968 and her master's degree in biochemistry in 1971. She completed certificates in metabolic and structural biochemistry, organic chemistry, physicochemical and molecular biology, and analytical chemistry.

In 1971 she began work as a researcher at the Pasteur Institute in Paris, while she was working on her *docteur ès sciences*, the equivalent in France of a Ph.D., which she completed in 1974. By 1975, at the age of 28, she had embarked on her career in science as assistant researcher at the Institute of National Health and Medical Research, with an affiliation with the Pasteur Institute. Also, from 1975–1976, she studied in the United States on a National Science Foundation grant to study methodology at the

National Institutes of Health (NIH) in Bethesda, Maryland. There she worked with Robert Gallo, who would again become a factor later in her career.

During these years Françoise met Claude Barré, a sound engineer, whom she married October 7, 1978. Rather than change her name to her new husband's, as her mother had, she hyphenated his with her father's, retaining both identities.

As early as 1971, Barré-Sinoussi began working on the retrovirus, now one of the best known viral families. Completely unknown prior to 1960, the retrovirus family comprises a group of viruses that have an odd way of going about their business—they "work backwards." While they vary in small ways, they all have one *modus operandi* in common: They insert their innards into the cytoplasm of the cells they infect and then they set about performing an incredible process—the behavior that gives them their name. Each virus carries onboard a single strand of RNA, plus an enzyme that enables it to use the RNA, instead of DNA, as a template to manufacture a complementary strand of DNA. This strand then becomes a template for creating a second copy of itself. Now the virus has a double-stranded DNA molecule, in double-helix form, the same form as the infected cell—instead of the RNA that these viruses usually have. Then the viral DNA just intrudes itself on the cell's DNA and camps there—no one is sure exactly how. From here on the behavior differs from one retrovirus to another. From within the DNA the virus may change the way the cell functions. It may replicate more viruses. It may cause the cell to replicate itself erratically, causing cancer. The possibilities are varied and no one is quite sure what triggers them. But because the infected cell looks so much like a normal cell, the retrovirus tends to throw the immune system off guard, and confuse it.

In 1971, at the age of 24, Barré-Sinoussi had started out working on retrovirus replication and expression in rats and mice, and her Ph.D. work for the next three years focused on developing anti-retroviral drugs that could block leukemia and sarcoma viruses from developing in mice. (One of these drugs later became used in therapeutic trials in AIDS patients.)

By 1979, Robert Gallo at the NIH had found a human retrovirus, which he called HTLV, for "human T-cell lymphoma virus," but he had a hard time convincing people that he had really found a human retrovirus, or that it was associated with T-cell malignancies, as he claimed. Gallo's flamboyant style, combined with jealousies about the big-money funding received by the NIH, led to strong skepticism. But because Gallo associated HTLV with cancers, when the AIDS epidemic broke out with all of its related cancers he immediately began to think in terms of a retrovirus, maybe even an HTLV virus, as its probable cause.

Meanwhile, by late 1982, several researchers in Paris—some of them at the Pasteur Institute—began to think along the same lines. Luc Montagnier, chief of the viral-oncology unit, had been working on retroviruses, but on another facet. Then he received a specimen taken from a swollen lymph node from a young French homosexual. It occurred to him that the patient could be in the early stages of AIDS. Was it an HTLV virus?

As Montagnier later recalled, "This was the beginning of excitement for us. Now there were two things to do: one was to maintain the virus, the other was to characterize it to see if it was an HTLV-like virus."

By this time Françoise Barré-Sinoussi, who was adjunct-chief of the department of virology, had been working on retroviruses for years and had developed expertise in the methods for isolating a virus from an infected blood cell. So when Montagnier began to think about retroviruses in connection with AIDS, he naturally turned to her, along with another colleague, Jean-Claude Chermann.

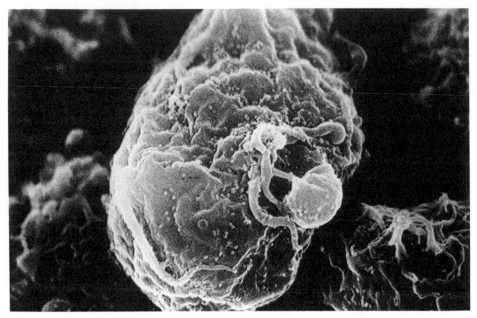

The AIDS virus   (Courtesy of the Centers for Disease Control, Atlanta, Georgia)

But the Pasteur researchers needed reagents—antibodies known to react against HTLV—so they could see what kind of virus they had. If the antibodies went after their virus, it was HTLV. Otherwise, if no reaction occurred, their virus was something else. So Montagnier asked Gallo to supply the reagents, which Gallo did.

In the meantime, Gallo had assembled a team in Bethesda to search for the AIDS virus. He knew he had the technology, the best available expertise, and the determination necessary. He felt sure it was just a matter of time until he came up with the virus.

But Françoise Barré-Sinoussi, Luc Montagnier, and Jean-Claude Chermann stole his thunder. In an article published in the May 1983 issue of the journal *Science*, with Barré-Sinoussi as lead author, the researchers gave an account of what they had found. When they had tested their virus with Gallo's HTLV reagents, no reaction had occurred. The HTLV antibodies didn't recognize their virus. It was something different, something new. As they explained in the article, it was "a retrovirus belonging to the family of recently discovered human T-cell leukemia viruses (HTLV), but clearly distinct from each previous isolate." Furthermore, they recounted, it had been "isolated from a Caucasian patient with signs and symptoms that often precede the acquired immune deficiency syndrome (AIDS)." But the Pasteur scientists were unwilling to jump to conclusions for which they didn't have strong evidence. They had used only one patient, and he probably had AIDS, but even that was uncertain. They wrote: "We tentatively conclude that this virus, as well as all previous HTLV isolates, belong to a family of T-lymphotropic retroviruses that . . . may be involved in several pathological syndromes, including AIDS."

In the same issue, however, Gallo had two articles announcing that he had found the HTLV virus in AIDS patients. But he hadn't actually isolated an AIDS virus yet. Meanwhile, the Pasteur group was having trouble growing a culture of their virus. Barré-Sinoussi and her colleagues felt sure they had isolated the AIDS virus. But the rest of the world remained skeptical. So, partly to convince former colleagues in the United States, Barré-Sinoussi sent samples of the virus to Gallo. Unfortunately, that was the beginning of a controversial scandal that ensued for the next 12 years.

Gallo's lab didn't have any luck either, and he had found a new virus of his own that they also had trouble growing in culture—the virus kept killing off the cells it infected. His lab

"We tentatively conclude that this virus . . . belong(s) to a family . . . that may be involved in several pathological syndromes, including AIDS."

—Barré-Sinoussi, Montagnier, and Chermann in their May 1983 *Science* article was used to the HTLV virus that caused cells to multiply, and they didn't recognize the new virus's cytopathology (tendency to kill cells) for what it was—an indication that they had the real thing.

Finally, in an effort to grow a culture, an assistant at the NIH lab made a soup of the viruses and succeeded in growing a culture. By January 1984, Gallo was sure he'd found the virus and he published his results in the May 1984 issue of *Science*. Margaret Heckler, at that time the U.S. Secretary of Health and Human Services, called a press conference to announce Gallo's success.

Montagnier was outraged. Part of the problem was that Gallo had publicly insulted the Pasteur team's science at a presentation Montagnier had made a few months earlier at Cold Spring Harbor Laboratories in New York. Secondly, he had slighted the Pasteur researchers' results in his account published in *Science*. But matters got worse.

A patent for an AIDS test based on Gallo's work was issued in 1985. The test established whether an individual's bloodstream contained antibodies to the AIDS virus—which did not necessarily mean the illness had been contracted. But it did mean that individual had been exposed. The availability of this test provided a great step forward in the effort to control the disease.

But researchers at the Pasteur Institute had uneasy feelings about this test. To them, it seemed likely that the development of the test was based, not on Gallo's original research, but on the AIDS virus they had isolated and provided samples of! By December, the Pasteur Institute had sued the United States to establish its own claim to discovery of the deadly virus, prior to the American researchers. Depositions, investigations, and ethics hearings followed in an agonizing sequence of events.

Barré-Sinoussi kept as far from all this pandemonium as possible. She focused on her scientific research, and she didn't get caught up in the brouhaha. She also managed to maintain good relations with her American colleagues and succeeded in continuing the exchange of information so vital in science. Consistently careful and professional, she tried to keep the media from running away with half-baked news whenever she had the opportunity. In early 1987, the Pasteur Institute announced that Jean-Claude Chermann had carried out a test to see if a widely sold French spermicide would kill the AIDS virus. In his report Chermann indicated that yes, a component of the Pharmatex spermacide had been shown to kill an AIDS virus in the laboratory.

But, speaking as a member of Chermann's team, Barré-Sinoussi emphasized the limitations of the test. Always concerned lest people should become overly confident about such an announcement, she warned that the result "must be taken very cautiously. We have not shown that the product, at the moment, prevents the transmission of AIDS in man." As she pointed out, "What we have shown is simply that when the HIV virus was mixed in a test tube with the Pharmatex product, the virus was killed, was inactivated, that it was then unable to infect white cells, lymphocytes, in vitro, in a test tube."

By 1988, Françoise Barré-Sinoussi's team was comparing parallel strains of the HIV virus—one capable of destroying its victim in a very short span of time, and one whose host has succeeded in defending against it without treatment. From such comparisons, she and her colleagues, working on the cutting edge of AIDS research, have been developing strategies for combating the disease. She described the work at a 1988 AIDS conference in Chicago, explaining that she and her colleagues had found that studying strains of the virus that produce unusual patterns of disease "are illuminating our understanding of HIV." To show what she meant, she described these two atypical case histories that they had tracked.

In the first, she and her team had tried to isolate the virus from a man from Zaire who had AIDS. To their surprise, they found that the virus killed culture cells in which it normally grows. The isolated virus seemed to cause disease much more rapidly than usual, and the man died very quickly. The same virus infected his wife, who also became ill, and so did her lover. Both died within three years—a much shorter time than the usual delay of five to eight years between infection and development of AIDS.

Barré-Sinoussi's team called this virus strain from Zaire HIV-NDK. When they examined it further, they discovered that it was 100 to 1,000 times more deadly to cells than the standard strain of HIV. They also found in tests that HIV-NDK exhibited many variations in the structure of the envelope protein on the surface of the virus, and this also distinguished it from viruses isolated from the United States and Europe. On the other hand, the envelope protein had close similarities to another strain of HIV isolated from another person from Zaire.

Generally, Barré-Sinoussi explained, viruses isolated from patients from Central Africa seemed to be more capable of killing cells than those found in the United States and Europe. And she extrapolated that the key might be a different gene for the envelope protein, explaining that "the biological properties of this virus may be related to the envelope gene itself."

In another case, said Barré-Sinoussi, a man developed acute encephalopathy, also known as AIDS dementia. During his illness, cerebrospinal fluid was drawn, from which the researchers in her team succeeded in isolating an AIDS virus. But, strangely, they were unable to find any trace of it in the lymphocytes in his blood. Then, in an unusually fortunate turn of events, the patient completely recovered spontaneously, without treatment of any kind. Even further mysterious, once he had recovered, Barré-Sinoussi's team could no longer isolate the virus either from his cerebrospinal

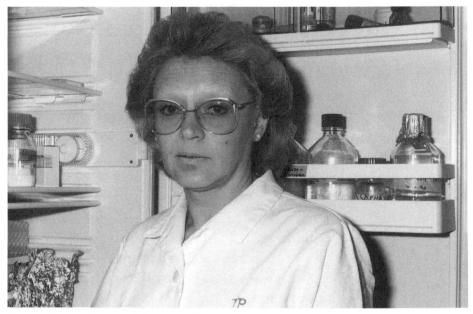

Barré-Sinoussi in her lab at the Pasteur Institute   (Courtesy of the Institut Pasteur)

fluid or from his blood. Antibodies did remain, however, in both fluids, presenting reinforcing evidence that the virus had been active in the man's system.

While studying the biological properties of the virus taken from this patient, Barré-Sinoussi and her team found that they couldn't grow it in the blood cells that HIV usually grows readily in. They could only grow the virus in immature cells, such as bone marrow cells. Barré-Sinoussi hypothesized that this case could provide a useful example of an individual whose natural defenses had succeeded in containing the infection.

Barré-Sinoussi is typically cautious and skeptical about all claimed advances, expecting proof before she thinks excitement is justified—the soundest scientific position to take. Has the experiment been checked and rechecked? Is it reproducible in other labs? These are the kinds of criteria that must be met. In a field like AIDS research, her stance is especially admirable, since a breakthrough is so desperately sought after and fame will certainly follow anyone who succeeds. And for the same reason, because the press and its readers and listeners jump so swiftly to unsound conclusions, caution is far more ethical.

In 1993, a colleague of Barré-Sinoussi's at the Pasteur Institute called a press conference to present the status of his research team's work on understanding how the AIDS virus infects a healthy cell. The atmosphere was charged. Gallo and other American researchers were present, looking skeptical (the ongoing controversy between the labs was still not settled), and the researcher was offended.

"While I was talking," he later told reporters, "Gallo was sitting in the front row laughing all the time."

But Barré-Sinoussi was unswayed by the political rivalries. As always, she was cautious and even-handed, commenting to reporters only, "It is a very interesting paper." Then she added a further caveat, "The danger is that whenever there is something interesting in this field, it gets blown out of proportion. . . . The problem is that these are preliminary data."

Françoise Barré-Sinoussi is the author and coauthor of more than 229 articles and publications, and her skill as a scientist has been recognized worldwide. She has received numerous honors for her work, including the Kôrber Foundation Award for the Promotion of European Science (1986), the French Academy of Medicine Award (1988), and the King Fayçal Prize in Medicine (from Saudi Arabia, 1993). She has also been named a knight of the French Order of Merit. Barré-Sinoussi's key participation in the discovery of the AIDS virus is recognized throughout the world, and she continues her work at the Pasteur Institute on projects she hopes will lead to other breakthroughs in the fight against this dread disease, as well as others.

In January 1994, Barré-Sinoussi was finally drawn into the Gallo-Montagnier controversy about which team discovered the AIDS virus first, and who should own the patent for the test. By now, U.S. federal science fraud investigators had opened up a separate case against Gallo for unethical scientific conduct. At this time, under oath, Barré-Sinoussi recounted that Gallo's former chief virologist, Mikulas Popovic, had confided to her in 1992 that he had intentionally pooled the sample of virus from the Pasteur lab with blood cells from American AIDS patients "to enhance the growth capacity of the virus." This, finally, was one of the most conclusive pieces of evidence against Gallo's insistence that there could not have been any contamination. After several false conclusions, in July 1995, the Gallo-Montagnier conflict came to an end. Gallo finally admitted that the virus used in the manufacture of the American AIDS test is the same virus Pasteur scientists sent to Gallo for analysis in 1983.

In May 1995, Gallo had already resigned his post as head of the National Cancer Institute at the NIH. The 12-year struggle was an unfortunate chapter in the history of the fight against disease—absorbing energies and talents that would have been far better spent finding out more about the AIDS virus, developing a vaccine against AIDS, and working on therapies for AIDS patients.

At the end of 1995, the hope for answers to the AIDS epidemic remained guarded. Reports indicated that the number of people infected with the AIDS virus continued to rise worldwide, with especially sharp increases in Africa and Southeast Asia.

"The consequences [of the Gallo-Pasteur dispute] for HIV research were severely damaging, leading, in part, to a corpus of scientific papers polluted with systematic exaggerations and outright falsehoods of unprecedented proportions."

—From the U.S. House of Representatives Investigative Report, January 1995

In 1993, scientists confirmed that the antiviral drug AZT provided no long-term benefit after all in delaying the onset of AIDS symptoms and eventual death. And Jonas Salk reported at a conference in 1993 that the use of one of his final products, an experimental AIDS vaccine on which much hope had been focused, had not slowed the course of the disease or lessened its severity.

However, with the conflict between France and the United States behind them, Barré-Sinoussi and her colleagues at the Pasteur Institute have been free again to focus on the science of finding answers, a job for which they have already amply shown their qualifications.

Chronology

July 30, 1947	Françoise Claire Sinoussi born in Paris
1975	Sinoussi joins Inserm (the French National Institute of Health and Medical Research) as an assistant researcher
1978	Sinoussi marries Claude Barré
1983	As part of a team headed by Luc Montagnier at the Pasteur Institute, Barré-Sinoussi isolates the virus that causes AIDS
1985	The Pasteur Institute files suit against the United States to establish the Pasteur claim that it discovered the AIDS virus prior to American researchers
1986	Sinoussi becomes Research Director at Inserm; receives the Kôrber Foundation Award for the Promotion of European Science
1988	Receives the Award of the French Academy of Medicine

1993   Becomes Chief of the Retrovirus Biology
Unit at the Pasteur Institute; receives the
King Fayçal Prize in Medicine (from
Saudi Arabia)

Further Reading

Chicago Tribune, 12/14/85, 1/14/87.

Barré-Sinoussi, F., *et al.* "Isolation of a T-lymphotropic retrovirus from a patient at risk for acquired immune deficiency syndrome (AIDS)." *Science*, 1983, 220, 868–871.

Crewdson, John. *Chicago Tribune*, 5/5/91, 9/15/91, 6/6/93, 1/19/94, 6/9/94, 6/19/94, 7/12/94, 12/22/94, 1/1/95, 5/25/95.

Fettner, Anne Giudici. *The Science of Viruses*. New York: Quill/William Morrow, 1990.

Fultz, Patricia N., Peter Nara, Françoise Barré-Sinoussi, Agnes Chaput, Michael L. Greenberg, Elizabeth Muchmore, Marie-Paule Kieny and Marc Girard. "Vaccine protection of chimpanzees against challenge with HIV-1-infected peripheral blood mononuclear cells." *Science*, June 19, 1992, p. 1687.

Hooper, Judith. "Interview: Paul Ewald." *Omni*, March 1995.

Kingman, Sharon. "AIDS Monitor: Unusual strains provide clues to the biology of the virus." *New Scientist*, 5/26/88, p. 41.

Levine, Arnold J. *Viruses*. New York: Scientific American Library, 1992.

Radetsky, Peter. *The Invisible Invaders: Viruses and the Scientists Who Pursue Them*. Boston: Little, Brown and Company, 1994.

Wain-Hobson, Simon, Jean-Pierre Vartanian, Michel Henry, Nicole Chenciner, Rémi Cheynier, Sylvie Delassus, Livia Pedroza Martins, Monica Sala, Marie-Thérèse Nugeyre, Denise Guétard, David Klatzmann, Jean-Claude Gluckman, Willy Rozenbaum, Françoise Barré-Sinoussi, and Luc Montagnier. "LAV revisited: origins of the early HIV-1 isolates from Institut Pasteur." *Science*, May 17, 1991, p. 961.

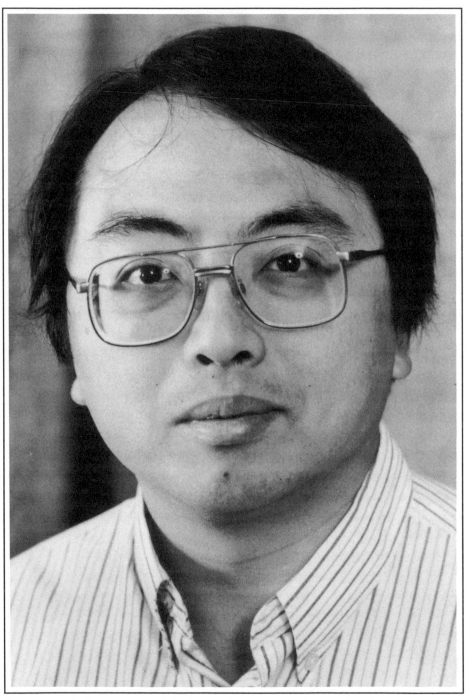

Lap-Chee Tsui (Courtesy of the Hospital for Sick Children, University of Toronto)

Lap-Chee Tsui

DISCOVERY OF THE CYSTIC FIBROSIS GENE (1950–)

Security was tight at the laboratory of Lap-Chee Tsui [Anglicized as choy] in Toronto during the summer of 1989. After a long, hard seven-year search, it looked like they had something. But they had to be sure. Was it really the right gene? Was the mutation they had found really linked to cystic fibrosis? Or was it just an odd coincidence?

"It's not a simple thing, where you say 'Eureka!' and go out and celebrate," Tsui commented later. It had to be certain. The 20 or so people who worked in the crowded, cheerful lab were used to working late. Now there was anticipation in the air as they geared up for even longer hours than usual. They had found a clue. But new experiments lay ahead, and meticulous testing. They had to check and recheck their results to prove they had found the right one.

Finally they were sure. On August 24, 1989, news conferences were called in Toronto and Washington, D.C. to announce the resolution to one of the great medical mysteries of the 20th century: Tsui, with his team at the Hospital for Sick Children in Toronto, and Francis Collins of the Howard Hughes Medical Institute at the University of Michigan had found the cause of cystic fibrosis, a frequently fatal disease that afflicts 30,000 people in North America alone.

Lap-Chee Tsui was born December 21, 1950, in Shanghai, China, but grew up in Hong Kong, where he lived in a small rural village on the outskirts of the city. There he developed his interest in nature, biology, and science in general, playing for hours as a boy in the nearby creeks and ponds. He caught tadpoles and goldfish, or watched closely as they went about their normal life in the water. He and his friends once raised a silkworm through its life cycle. They stripped leaves from nearby trees to feed it (much to the annoyance of the tree's owner). And they watched it spin its cocoon of silk, later to emerge as a moth and fly away.

Tsui attended college at the Chinese University in Hong Kong, where he received both his bachelor's and master's degrees in biology. At this time, his greatest interest was molecular biology. He traveled to the United States, to the University of Pittsburgh in Pennsylvania, where he completed his doctoral work from 1974 to 1979, training under Roger Hendrix. In his doctoral thesis, which was primarily on molecular biology, Tsui explored the structure and morphogenesis of a simple organism, a virus that infects bacteria, to look at some of the basic mechanisms in its life processes. The following year, as he concluded a brief postdoctoral stint working with retroviruses in the Biology Division at the Oak Ridge National Laboratory in Tennessee, he heard that Jack Riordan and Manuel Buchwald were looking for a postdoctoral fellow to help them probe the causes of cystic fibrosis at the Hospital for Sick Children, University of Toronto, Ontario.

Toronto, he thought, was a good place to go. (Certainly a lot less humid than Tennessee.) Working on a disease like cystic fibrosis attracted him—it was a worthy mission. And genetics could be an interesting tool. He became interested, read everything he could find on the subject, and applied.

That was 1981, and he was right, it was a good place to go and he has been there ever since. Now a Canadian citizen, Tsui is a professor in the Department of Molecular and Medical Genetics and holds the Sellers Chair in Cystic Fibrosis Research at the Hospital for Sick Children. He and his wife make their home in the Toronto area and have two sons.

Looking back on his graduate and postgraduate years, Tsui once described three major professional influences in his life to Barry Shell, a Canadian writer: First, he said, was K. K. Mark, in Hong Kong, "who taught me to concentrate on a single thing and be good at it." Second was Roger Hendrix, in Pittsburgh, "who gave me the freedom to do my own thing and was very supportive of whatever I did." Third, was Manuel Buchwald, in Toronto, who "taught me how to be critical and look at the broader perspective."

A fourth important influence in his life was a man he called his "uncle" although he is no relation, an older man he met in Pittsburgh, Dr. Han Chang. Tsui said Han Chang taught him "to be more flexible and to be adaptive and to look at things broadly." Most important, he taught him the importance of playing by the rules of the game, which shift depending upon whether the game is basketball or soccer. Or depending

"He taught me to be more flexible and to be adaptive and to look at things broadly."

—Lap-Chee Tsui

upon where you're playing—in Hong Kong, Pittsburgh, or Toronto.

In 1985, together with Manuel Buchwald and other scientists, Tsui identified the first DNA marker linked to CF on chromosome 7, one of the 23 pairs of chromosomes contained in every human cell. Four years later, Tsui led the team of researchers at the Hospital for Sick Children and University of Michigan to "a major breakthrough in human genetics"—they succeeded in isolating the defective gene responsible for cystic fibrosis and defining the principal mutation. The result of seven years of intensive research, Tsui's achievement was described in *Science* as "the most refreshing scientific development of 1989" and hailed that same year in Canada's *Maclean's* Honor Roll as one of the "discoveries of hope at the heart of human life."

The attraction of this work, for Tsui, is understanding the structure and function of genes, especially genes that are involved in disease. By understanding the processes, Tsui reasons, he can be more helpful in treating diseases. Cystic fibrosis is particularly compelling, since it is the most common inherited fatal disease among Caucasians, occurring about once in every 2,500 births. Although many CF patients now live to be 20 or 30 years old through the use of antibiotics and other physical therapy, up to a few years ago, most CF patients died in childhood. If both parents carry the gene responsible for the disease, they have a one-in-four chance of having an affected child.

The technique Tsui and his team used to find the gene is called positional cloning, also referred to as reverse genetics, or positional analysis. Genes contain the blueprints that tell cells how to make proteins, the chemicals that make up all living tissue and regulate body functions. But if geneticists don't know about the specific function

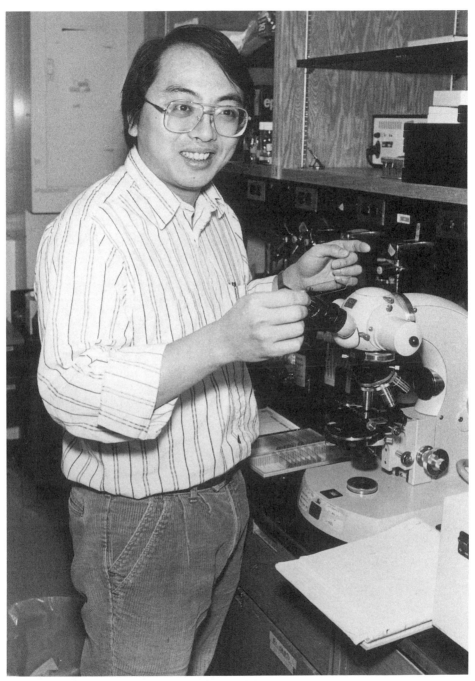

Tsui in his lab at the Hospital for Sick Children in Toronto (Courtesy of the Hospital for Sick Children, University of Toronto)

of the gene they're looking for, and don't know what protein it encodes, they usually have to use positional cloning to find it.

In cystic fibrosis, the exocrine glands secrete abnormally thick mucus, which often causes obstruction of the pancreas and chronic infections of the lungs. From observation of patterns, it became obvious that the disorder is transmitted genetically from parents to child via a recessive gene. That is, to contract the disease a child would have to inherit the gene from both parents. But no one knew exactly what the mechanism was that caused the disease. So positional cloning, a complex process of analysis based on mapping and linkage analysis, became the logical approach. Tsui's team knew that the CF gene was located on chromosome 7, and a link had been shown between CF and the longest of the chromosome's two arms. But finding the gene wasn't easy. No previous study had turned up any clues. Ultimately, the procedure was tedious and exacting.

First, they cloned a portion of chromosome 7 that they knew must include the CF gene. Then they cloned overlapping portions of the chromosome in a complicated process made more difficult because the overlapping had to be done sequentially. Problems sometimes develop in stepping through a chromosome region as long as the one they were investigating. That's where Collins came in, using a technique called "jumping clones," at which he was expert. Finally, they found a large gene, 230,000 bases in length, in which three deletions occurred—three nucleotides that code for a particular amino acid, three beads that should have been on the necklace but were missing. It was May 1989. They had found a mutation. But was the gene the right one—the one that caused CF?

Then the checking began. They examined a large number of DNAs from CF patients, looking for the same deletions.

They found that 70 percent of the CF chromosomes among the North American patients tested had the same mutation. These were compared to normal chromosomes from parents of affected children: They did not show the mutation.

Other mutations have also been found in the same gene among CF patients—some 600 different kinds of mutations by 1996—accounting for the other 30% of the patients whose genes did not show the first mutation. By 1996, the evidence was overwhelming.

During the summer of 1989, while Tsui and Collins worked to authenticate the gene (seeking to prove the Tsui lab had found the right one), Riordan isolated the protein that it normally makes in healthy individuals. The protein functions as a kind of "gate" to regulate the amount of chloride, sodium, and water in cells lining the respiratory and digestive tracts. The researchers dubbed this gate CFTR (an inexact acronym for "cystic fibrosis transmembrane conductance regulator"). In normal individuals, water moistens the airways, diluting the mucus in much the same way that paint thinner makes paint runnier. But in cystic fibrosis, the regulating protein is defective. Some of the 1,480 amino acids normally in the gene either aren't there or aren't quite right. So the protein isn't produced exactly right and it doesn't do its job. As a result, chloride and sodium build up in abnormal concentrations in the cells. By osmosis, the chloride and sodium draw water from the surface of the airways into the cells, leaving mucus in the respiratory tract thick and sticky.

Tsui and his colleagues continue to explore the effect produced by the loss of function of CFTR in the biology of the intestine, reproductive organs, and lungs. In particular, they are looking at how CFTR is regulated and expressed in both humans and rodents.

Knowing the architecture of the CF protein and how it works will permit drug designers to create new drugs, much as Gertrude Elion did, specifically engineered to correct the fault in the cellular function. Having the CF gene in hand also enables geneticists to screen for CF in families where the disease has been known to occur. And the CF gene discovery has raised high hopes for gene therapy as well.

In September 1995, however, discouraging results came in from a carefully controlled study of gene therapy for cystic fibrosis at the University of North Carolina at Chapel Hill School of Medicine. Researchers tried squirting aerosol concoctions into the nose passages, windpipes, and, in some cases, lungs of patients suffering from CF. But these weren't ordinary aerosols. The aerosols contained genetically engineered viruses, called adenoviruses, to transfer normal genes to these areas, which are directly affected by CF. Reports coming in during 1993 had seemed to show the strategy was working well in nasal passages and only needed to be applied to lung tissue, which is more critical but harder to reach. Now, in the Chapel Hill study, the adenovirus "ferry" appeared to fail.

But researchers in the field have not become discouraged. The technology is new—only five years old—and still crude. Refinements and more sophisticated approaches promise to pay off in the future.

Gene therapy, still in its infancy, continues to hold promise in the battle against a host of deadly diseases, including AIDS, cancer, and atherosclerosis. And for CF, Dr. Claude Lenfant, director of the U.S. National Heart, Lung, and Blood Institute declared, "We are confident

> "We are confident that gene therapy will someday provide a cure for CF."
>
> —Claude Lenfant, director of the U.S. National Heart, Lung, and Blood Institute, 1995

that gene therapy will someday provide a cure for CF. Significant advances hinge on this crucial interplay between 'bench and bedside' research."

Meanwhile, Tsui and his team continue their work. Tsui has established a worldwide consortium of about 130 different laboratories that are working on CF in 30 different countries. The first of its kind, the consortium communicates informally by newsletter and fax, and has become a model for similar groups studying genetic disease. He is also working on other disease gene analyses, including the mapping of the gene for Tourette syndrome, and he is a key participant in the effort to map the human genome, in particular the physical mapping study of chromosome 7. He is active in coordinating the Canadian Genetic Disease Network, a nation-wide program supported by the Federal government of Canada to promote implementation of research results in the private sector.

Lap-Chee Tsui has been named Scientist (1989–1994) and Senior Scientist (1995–2000) of the Medical Research Council of Canada, Fellow of the Royal Society of Canada, Fellow of the Royal Society of London, and Member of Academia Sinica. In addition to many national and international awards, he has received honorary doctoral degrees from University of King's College, University of New Brunswick, St. Francis Xavier University (Antigonish, Nova Scotia), and the Chinese University of Hong Kong. He was inducted into the Order of Canada (Officer rank) in 1991.

But for Tsui, who devotes most of his spare time to volunteer work in the Chinese community, science is for everyone. The disciplines are tough, he admits. But knowing physics and biology, he believes, knowing how things work, can enrich your life. "Basically," he likes to say, "science is a foundation for genuine common sense."

Chronology

December 21, 1950	Lap-Chee Tsui is born in Shanghai
1972	Receives B.S. in biology at the Chinese University of Hong Kong
1974	Earns M.Phil. in biology at the Chinese University of Hong Kong
1979	Receives Ph.D. from the University of Pittsburgh (Pennsylvania)
1979–1980	Serves as postdoctoral investigator, Biology Division, Oak Ridge National Laboratory, Oak Ridge, Tennessee
1981–1983	Works as postdoctoral fellow, Department of Genetics, Hospital for Sick Children, Toronto, Ontario
1985	Tsui and colleagues at the Hospital for Sick Children identify the first DNA marker linked to cystic fibrosis (CF) on chromosome 7
1989	Tsui leads a team that succeeds in isolating the defective gene responsible for CF and defining the principal mutation (ΔF508)
1992	Becomes chair of Chromosome 7 Committee, Genome Data Base Project

Further Reading

Buchwald, Manuel. "Isolation of the Cystic Fibrosis Gene," in *Canadian Health Research: A Salute to Excellence*. Westmount, Quebec: Canadians for Health Research, 1992.

McConkey, Edwin H. *Human Genetics: the Molecular Revolution*. Boston: Jones and Bartlett Publishers, 1993.

Shell, Barry. *Great Canadian Scientists Project*, Wide World Web site: http://fas.sfu.ca/css/gcs

Chicago Tribune, 10/10/85, 8/24/89, 8/25/89, 2/1/90, 9/28/95.

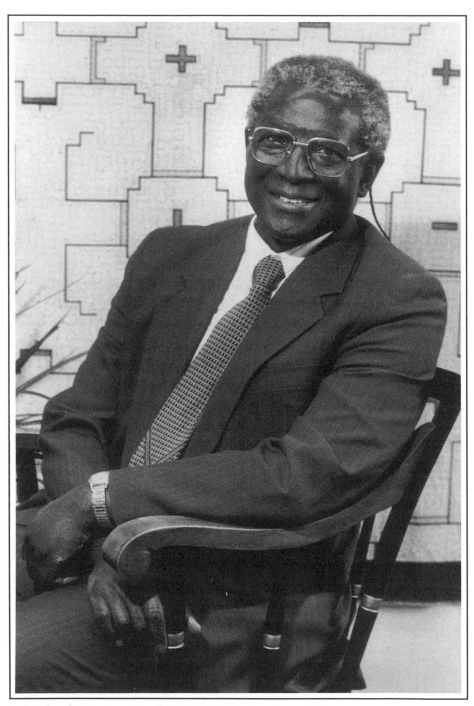

Adetokunbo Lucas (Copyright © 1995 by Sue Owrutsky)

Adetokunbo Lucas

THE FIGHT FOR
WORLD HEALTH (1931–)

M ore than 95 million people make their home in the Federal Republic of Nigeria, the most populous country in Africa. It is a land of many contrasts. Its large urban areas—Lagos, on the coast, a city of 1.3 million; and Ibadan, a few hundred miles inland, with a population of 1.2 million—bustle with commerce and manufacturing, the site of pharmaceutical and automobile factories, as well as scientific institutes, universities, and libraries. Yet these areas strain under the rapidly growing population, which frequently faces power failures, water supply interruptions, and traffic jams. In Lagos, water pollution has become a serious problem, as well as atmospheric pollution.

Having a land mass of 356,669 square miles, about the size of Texas and Kansas together, Nigeria is located on the west coast of Africa, just south of the Sahara Desert. It has few high elevations, but a wide range in rainfall levels and vegetation, from savanna and even high desert in the north to the rain forest belt in the south.

In the savanna, the change of seasons is most pronounced, with varied climates, typified by the long, often very hot dry season when water is scarce. Except for the plains around the city of Kano, where the population density is high, people in the savanna don't have to deal with the health problems presented by crowded conditions. Farmers keep on the move during the dry season when little farming can be done, and pastoral nomadic groups also move over large areas to find pasture for their flocks and herds of cattle. But the people in these regions live exposed to the hazards of water shortage, excessive heat, hunger, and even famine.

On the other hand, in parts of eastern Nigeria, the rain falls in torrents, as much as 400 inches a year. There, the humidity is high, and the temperature remains moderate throughout the year. In the forests and rainy regions, however, lurk other hazards—including disease-carrying insects and parasites, high population density, and conditions conducive to the spread of infectious disease. These are among the areas where Burkitt found the lymphoma later associated with the Epstein-Barr virus.

This varied country—with its many contrasting health challenges—is the land that Adetokunbo Lucas calls home, and it is where he first began his practice of medicine, just as Nigeria was gaining independence, in 1960.

Adetokunbo (Ade) Olumide Oluwole Lucas was born November 25, 1931 into a family where education was highly regarded. His father, J. Olumide Lucas, who held a doctor of divinity (D.D.) degree from Dunelm, became a clergyman in the Episcopal Church. He also had a keen interest in traditional religions of West Africa and Egypt, an avocation he pursued with a level of academic and scholarly intensity that few people apply even to their chosen professions. "On Sunday he would preach in church," his son later recalled, "and then the rest of the week he would study traditional religious customs and beliefs."

Lucas grew up with lots of good role models—"lots and lots of uncles," as he puts it. His father was one of seven children, and his mother, R. Ibironke Oluwole, grew up in a family of six. Some of Ade's uncles were lawyers, and he sometimes daydreamed as a child of becoming a "hanging judge," but that, he says, is like saying you're going to be a fireman when you grow up. When it really came down to choosing a career, he had no hesitation. He would become a physician, like his favorite uncle, his mother's older brother, who trained in Scotland and became a medical officer of health in Lagos. Another key figure in his youth was his mother's younger sister's husband, who also trained in Scotland and became the first director of medical services in Nigeria, before independence.

So Lucas took it for granted that he would follow the trail of his uncles and father to train academically in the United Kingdom and return to work in Nigeria. He received his basic medical training at the University of Durham in England, Queen's University in Ireland, and the London School of Hygiene and Tropical Diseases. Like his uncles, when he did return, he was drawn away from the attractive prospect of private practice. While he could have made an excellent income healing private patients, the bigger picture held a stronger appeal.

Freshly home from medical training in Dublin and London, Ade Lucas accepted a position in the teaching hospital at the newly forming University College in Ibadan. There, he was in for a shock. "The disease patterns in Nigeria turned out to be very different than what I'd expected," he later told a journalist. "According to the model I'd learned, Nigerian health problems should consist chiefly of diseases that were common all over the world, with the addition of parasitic diseases as the main variation. But I found that in Nigeria even heart disease and diabetes behaved very, very differently."

Although he had always enjoyed clinical work with patients and found it exciting, now he began to feel enormous frustration. "So many of the cases that came to us," he later explained, "shouldn't have happened at all." Youngsters would come in with the severe muscle spasms of tetanus, often on the verge of death, and the medical staff would be challenged with trying to save them. But these cases should never have happened. "They could have been prevented," said Lucas, "with a 10-cent immunization."

In 1963, he went to Boston to enter a two-year master's degree program in Hygiene at the Harvard School of Public Health. On his return to Nigeria, he served as chair of the Department of Preventive and Social Medicine at the University of Ibadan from 1965 to 1976 and chaired the Medical Research Council of Nigeria from 1973 to 1976.

That's when Lucas's focus shifted from cure to prevention. And to the larger picture—to the process of getting prevention to the people that needed it, through programs of public health and public health policy.

The World Health Organization in Geneva gave him a golden opportunity. They asked him to direct the newly established Special Program for Research and Training in Tropical Diseases in Geneva. Lucas was now in a position to make a difference internationally—to put to work everything he had learned about disease in the tropics, actual conditions, administration coordination, and overarching strategies for achieving effective results in worldwide public health.

Established two years earlier, this TDR (Tropical Disease Research) program had set out to stimulate research capability in developing countries on malaria and other diseases common to those areas. The problem was, as Lucas put it, a "geographical dislocation": Those who were capable of carrying out needed research were not located in the countries where the diseases were rampant. The traditional approach, following the model set by agricultural research programs, was to set up isolated research stations operating as nodes in the field, hoping to build a critical mass of research that would lead to solutions. But when Ade Lucas became head of the WHO Special Program in 1976, he tried another approach. He began to organize networks of cooperating scientists and institutions—within both developing and developed countries—to work on aspects of tropical disease research.

For the next 10 years, Lucas engineered the formation of networks involving more than 2,400 projects in some 100 countries. During the decade, the program was involved in the development of 50 new products ranging from new anti-malarial drugs to toxins for the control of insects that transmit infections.

At the outset of the program, Lucas brought a key group of scientists together, who reviewed the state of the art and identified the needs and the research needed to accomplish the goals. The group looked at the need to use available drugs in combination and monitor the impact. But this approach required sophisticated technology to monitor the results—technology not available in the areas where clinics were treating leprosy patients. For example, they needed immuno-suppressed mice to check the time it took to eradicate all residual traces of the bacillus that causes leprosy. So they set up collaborations between researchers in the United Kingdom and the United States and clinicians in India or Africa.

Each grantee became a research center. The grant didn't take him or

"We didn't have to hire and fire. We didn't have to keep dead wood."

—Ade Lucas, 1995

her away from the location where the greatest productivity was possible—the location where facilities and equipment were available, where experimental animals were already on hand. These scientific working groups worked in an effective and flexible way. As Lucas put it, "We didn't have to hire and fire. We didn't have to keep dead wood." And when researchers had completed the work funded by a grant, they could move on to other work. The approach was very cost-effective, bringing together experience from all over the world and coordinating it to produce the needed results. "We got all the people together on a small planet, but not in the same institution," Lucas quipped, recounting the story in 1995.

Of all the projects, Lucas was proudest of the research on chemotherapy for treatment of leprosy, although, he said, this actually may not be the most important achievement of the program. "It is the one I feel most happy about," he commented. At the beginning of the program, very little progress had been made against the incidence of leprosy for 20 to 30 years.

Found in many tropical areas, an estimated 10 million people suffer from leprosy, which is caused by the *Myobacterium leprae*. The disease affects the skin and superficial nerves and, left untreated, the lesions of leprosy can cause severe deformation, loss of sensation, paralysis, and gangrene.

One of the difficulties faced by leprosy researchers at the time the program began was that no one had ever succeeded in growing a culture of the leprosy bacillus. Tests had to be made on tissue samples scraped from lesions on human patients. The only other place researchers found where they could grow the bacillus was the foot pad of a mouse. It took nine months to develop a sample, and then, of course, because of the very small size of the mouse's foot pad, the quantity gained was minute.

Then the discovery was made at a lab in the southern United States that the leprosy bacillus could be grown in abundance on the 9-banded armadillo, although it took two years to develop. But how could you expect a scientist working in Germany first to learn how to keep an armadillo in a lab, then infect it with leprosy, and then wait two years to perform research on the resulting culture? So the TDR special program funded the establishment of a leprosy bacillus bank. Then they arranged for the production of bacilli from armadillos, produced by the lab that knew how to do it, at a marginal cost because it was just an extension of what the lab was already doing for their own research. This provided a source of top-grade leprosy bacilli—several kilograms stored in a deep freeze—that could be made available to researchers for doing studies. In this way, they were able to get a great deal of mileage out of very small grants.

The program's affiliation with WHO helped accomplish another goal: freedom from the encumbrances of politics and bureaucracy. All decisions were made by scientists instead of bureaucrats. And decisions were made using scientific criteria, not political ones. They avoided the pressures to apportion a balanced number of grants, country by country—so many to the UK, so many the United States, so many to Germany or France. They made the decisions based on who could do the job best.

The key researcher in the search for a drug against leprosy was located in Australia, where leprosy in humans is virtually nonexistent. He was a veterinary pathologist, and he had never even seen a case of human leprosy. But he was interested because leprosy was related to a problem ranchers were having with cattle in Australia. The program's review board determined, through the system of issuing requests for proposals, that this pathologist's laboratory was best equipped in terms of expertise and technology to do the job. A compound would be tested in London, and then in another research site. If it passed those tests, then it was sent to the "cattle screen." This screening test had the best predicted results, but of course it was very expensive because it involved infecting an otherwise healthy cow with leprosy. The search produced a tangible result: One compound turned out to be the most effective—ivermectin—and it is now available, requiring one dose a year. Now for the first time in many years, leprosy is in steady decline. In 1993, as the 20th anniversary of the founding of the TDR special program approached, WHO announced the goal of eradicating leprosy completely by 2000.

One of the program's less tangible legacies is that it brought many scientists into communication with each other who otherwise would never have talked. For example, it funded a physicist working for General Electric who had developed an interesting technique for detecting antigens. This interdisciplinary approach—also being used by Susumu Tonegawa and Lap-Chee Tsui in their research—is clearly the way of the future in science. It is a recognition of the enormous overlapping areas of method, data, and concepts in all fields.

By the end of the decade of work, the program had funded about 50 products, some minor, some significant, but most done through this collaborative effort of many teams, working closely with the private sector.

In the late 1980s, Lucas moved on to head the Carnegie Corporation of New York's Program on Strengthening Human Resources in Developing Countries. Turning his focus to a more particular problem that had always troubled him, Lucas supervised a program focused on the problem of maternal mortality. With the end goal of finding ways to encourage safe motherhood, especially in developing countries, he oversaw the funding of grants to stimulate research in many parts of the world. And he directed the organization of the first international conference on safe motherhood, which took place in Nairobi in 1987.

From 1990 to 1995, as professor of international health at the Harvard School of Public Health, Lucas directed the establishment of a series of seminars, known as the Harvard International Health Leadership Forum, designed to train ministers of public health. "It occurred to me" he said, "that everybody's having workshops except those at the top. Yet a minister of health may be just a successful politician" who suddenly finds himself in charge of the public health policy of an entire nation.

Three former ministers of public health served as resource people, and the forum workshops also provided a good interaction between the ministers of public health who attended and clinicians working in the field. Ironically, as Lucas indicated, those who make public health policy are often elected officials who may or may not have any background in public health. They may know the technology in their own area very well—perhaps neurosurgery or cardiology—but know little about broader public health policy issues. So the HIHLF workshop was designed to provide an "eye-opening" experience with a one-week intensive seminar. Most important of all, it took place in a non-threatening environment, providing a venue protected from the public eye. There the participants could ask what they might consider "stupid questions" they wouldn't want to be caught asking—but to which they needed answers.

The workshops have generally invited public health ministers from a group of countries in a geographical area, since they usually share similar challenges—one for Caribbean countries, one for West African countries, one for the new ministers of South Africa, one in the future for Asian countries. Bureaucrats were banned. The idea was to provide a closed meeting in which the ministers could confess what they didn't understand and where learning from colleagues could take place without loss of face. "I think everyone would get frightened," Lucas remarked, "if the newly elected minister of health admitted in public that he didn't know anything about public health policy." The Harvard setting has provided an academic learning situation, face to face with a few key resource people and clinicians. Here, asking and learning is the point. And no one is running a tape recorder or a TV camera. The process is private—and productive.

Lucas recounted one incident where the former minister of public health from an Asian country discussed some of the strategies he used for establishing new policies and programs for the production of pharmaceuticals in his country. As he explained at the workshop, first he had to mobilize the support of the medical profession, and then coordinate the pharmaceutical companies finally to gain the kind of cooperation that he needed. When he shared these ideas and strategies with ministers at his level from other countries, the result was some new insights about how to get the job done. At international meetings and conferences, according to Lucas, this kind of exchange rarely takes place because thousands of dollars in grants hang in the balance. No one ever wants to admit that things aren't going well or that obstacles are in the way of progress. No one ever wants to ask a stupid question. That would undercut that person's image and ability to command respect in his or her own country, and in some cases, it would damage the potential for gaining grants. The Harvard School of Public Health program provided an environment where real training could take place at a level that Lucas considers more important even than the hands-on level of the clinician.

"If a surgeon makes mistakes," he explained, "he'll kill two or three patients a day, with a total of maybe 100 to 300 a year. But if you have a lousy minister of public health making poor policy decisions, you're looking at thousands and thousands of deaths." Training neurosurgeons effectively is less important than training public health officers,

Lucas said, and yet millions of dollars of resources are put into training neurosurgeons and practically nothing into training public health officials.

Ade Lucas and his wife, the former Stella Norman-Williams, have four children, now scattered all over the world, and Lucas enjoys visiting them although he makes his home in Nigeria. Of two sons, one is a software engineer in Boston and the other a microcomputer analyst in London; and of two daughters, one is a systems programmer in Abidjan, Ivory Coast, and the other an agricultural biotechnician in Lagos, Nigeria.

In 1986, at Harvard's 350th anniversary celebration, Lucas was one of 20 alumni to receive the Harvard Medal. The citation reads, "Harvard salutes this champion of public health for his lifelong commitment to limiting tropical disease and combating ignorance in all people." He has received many other awards from institutions and professional groups, and in 1981 he was named Officer of the Order of the Federal Republic of Nigeria, a high national honor.

Adetokunbo Lucas has spent a lifetime putting a worldwide vision into effect: a vision of a healthier world through communication and effective cooperative effort. He has brought energy, expertise, compassion, and an overriding sense of humanity, dignity, and objectivity to the cause. Through teamwork, he has achieved some impressive results. And he has left a clear path for others to follow.

"If a surgeon makes mistakes, he'll kill two or three patients a day, with a total of maybe 100 to 300 a year. But if you have a lousy minister of public health making poor policy decisions, you're looking at thousands and thousands of deaths."

—Ade Lucas, 1995

Chronology

November 25, 1931	Adetokunbo Lucas is born in Nigeria
1953	Receives bachelor's degree in basic biomedical sciences, Durham University, England
1956	Receives bachelor's degree in medicine, bachelor's degree in surgery both with honors, Durham University
1959	Awarded diploma in public health, Queen's University, Belfast, Northern Ireland
1960	Awarded diploma of tropical medicine and hygiene, London School of Hygiene and Tropical Medicine
1964	Receives M.S., hygiene, Harvard School of Public Health, Boston, Massachusetts
1965–76	Serves as chair of the Department of Preventive and Social Medicine, University of Ibadan, Nigeria
1973–76	Chairs the Medical Research Council of Nigeria
1976–86	Directs the special program for research and training in tropical diseases of the World Health Organization, World Bank and UNDP, Geneva, Switzerland
1986	Receives the Harvard Medal
1986–90	Chairs the Carnegie program on strengthening human resources in developing countries
1991	Becomes chair of the advisory board of the Rockefeller Foundation's "Public Health Schools Without Walls" program

| 1990–1995 | Serves as Professor of International Health, Harvard School of Public Health |

Further Reading

Most of the material for this chapter came from interviews and unpublished sources. The main published sources are:

"International Courtships." *Around the School: News and Notices of the Harvard School of Public Health*, January 25, 1991, pp. 1–2.

Parry, E. H. O., editor. *Principles of Medicine in Africa*. Oxford, Nairobi, and Ibadan: Oxford University Press, 1976.

Epilogue

At the end of the 20th century, the road to worldwide health looks both more promising and bumpier than it did in 1950. The tools are better, the technology is improved, and we understand much more about the pathogens that cause disease and how the body fights them.

Macfarlane Burnet, Peter Medawar, and Susumu Tonegawa and others have helped us understand the immune system and how it works. Researchers like Rita Levi-Montalcini, Anthony Epstein, Lap-Chee Tsui, and Françoise Barré-Sinoussi have used insight, imagination, and high-tech tools to discover other basic facts about the process of disease, how the body functions, and how its enemies work. This understanding, in turn, provides insights for scientists like Jonas Salk and Albert Sabin as they develop vaccines, tests, and drugs. Meanwhile, Gertrude Elion and her colleagues in the pharmaceutical industry have given us better methods for developing medicines to fight specific diseases. From epidemiologists like Denis Burkitt we have gained new insights into how diseases spread and where and why. And policymakers like Ade Lucas and Bernard Kouchner have helped set aside political and national concerns to address the larger issues of human health and coordinate the fight.

Yet human health, we've discovered, is a moving target, not nearly so easily hit by the "silver bullets" of science as everyone believed at the beginning of the 20th century. As evolutionary biologist Paul Ewald of Amherst College pointed out, a disease organism's goal is to survive and produce more offspring than competing organisms. Those that multiply too fast or are too destructive tend to kill or immobilize their hosts before they can spread—and they become less prevalent just through natural selection. "Changes in circumstances," any circumstances, Ewald points out, including human behavior, "can shift a pathogen from mildness to virulence, or vice versa."

The fight against disease is a constantly shifting battle. And to gain ground consistently, both now and in the future, we'll have to martial all our intelligence, resources, and flexibility to keep that balance shifting in our favor. And so the fight continues—as humankind, with the aid of science, battles against disease. The call is out, as always, for new recruits, new fighters, and new weapons, in the laboratories and in the front lines. It is an age-old fight, one that will challenge all our resources far into the 21st century.

Index

This index is designed as an aid to access the narrative text and special features. Page numbers in **boldface** indicate key topics. Page numbers in *italic* indicate illustrations or captions. A "c" following the page number indicates chronology.